Mary R. Lunt

February 1972.

Viruses and Cancer

Viruses and Cancer

SIR CHRISTOPHER ANDREWES
MD, Ll.D, FRCP, FRS, FC Path.

49,078

WEIDENFELD AND NICOLSON
5 Winsley Street London W1

SBN 297 00218 X
Printed in Great Britain
by Richard Clay (The Chaucer Press), Ltd.,
Bungay, Suffolk

Contents

List of Plates   vii
Acknowledgments   viii
Preface   ix
1 Overgrowth and Cancer   1
2 The Viruses Involved   8
3 Fowl Tumours: Early History   12
4 Fowl Leukaemias   18
5 Defective Avian Tumour Viruses and 'Helpers'   27
6 Fowl Tumours in Other Species   32
7 Breast Cancer in Mice   39
8 Leukaemias in Mice   46
9 Leukaemias in Other Mammals   58
10 Some DNA-containing Tumour Viruses   63
11 Cell Transformation by DNA-Viruses   72
12 New Tumour Antigens   80
13 Warts in Rabbits and Other Species   85
14 Poxviruses   94
15 Tumours in Frogs and Fishes   99
16 Burkitt Tumours   104
17 Experiments on Synergism   112
18 Viral Oncolysis   122
19 More about Tumour Immunity   126
20 Unanswered Questions   132
   References   140
   Glossary   160
   Index   163

List of Plates

[*Between pages 86 and 87*]

1 Electron micrograph of herpes virions
2 Herpes-type intranuclear inclusion bodies
3 Leg of chick bearing a Rous sarcoma
4 Histological appearance of Rous sarcoma
5 'Pock' on chorio-allantoic membrane induced by Rous virus
6 Foci of cells in culture transformed by Rous virus
7 Chick paralysed by Marek's disease
8 Nerve of Marek-disease infected chick
9 Mouse with mammary tumour
10 Histological appearance of mammary tumour
11 Electron micrograph of C particles of Moloney leukaemic virus
12 Section through cheek-pouch of hamster inoculated with human mammary tumour
13 Rat with polyoma-induced kidney tumour
14 Electron micrograph of polyoma virions
15 Electron micrograph of adenovirus virion
16 Diagram of adenovirus virion
17 Warts on abdomen of rabbit
18 Carcinomatous change in rabbit warts
19 Section through a human wart
20 Lesions of jaagsiekte
21 Yaba virus growth on a monkey's face
22 Electron micrograph of molluscum contagiosum virus
23 Child with Burkitt tumour of the mandible
24 The same fourteen days after treatment

Acknowledgments

The author would like to thank the following for permission to reproduce photographs in this book: Mrs J. D. Almeida, plate 1; Dr J. A. Armstrong, plates 2, 11; Mrs C. Smith, plate 3; Dr R. J. C, Harris, plates 4, 10; Dr F. C. Chesterman, plate 5; Miss Carole Eveson, plate 6; Dr P. M. Biggs, plates 7, 8; Dr D. C. Roberts, plate 9; Dr F. C. Chesterman and the Royal College of Surgeons, plate 12; Dr F. C. Chesterman and CIBA foundation, plate 13; Drs G. D. Birnie and R. Dourmeashkin, plate 14; Dr H. G. Pereira, plates 15, 16; *Journal of experimental Medicine*, plate 17; Dr R. A. B. Drury, plate 19; Dr D. I. Nisbet, plate 20; *Nature*, plate 21; Dr R. Dourmeashkin, plate 22; Dr D. P. Burkitt and Springer-Verlag, plates 23, 24. The author would also like to thank Dr Miles Williams for permission to reproduce the climate map of Africa on page 105.

Preface

For several years there has been increasing interest in the role of viruses in causing tumours in some birds and mammals and in their possible importance in human cancers. Whether or not they are concerned in human cancer, their study has led to important extensions in our knowledge about the disease: of how viruses can lead to malignant changes in cells, and especially of the role of immunity in protection against cancer. The literature on the subject is vast and scattered, as is testified by the 370 or so selected references on pages 140 to 159. It has therefore seemed worth while to bring together the facts as we now know them. They are marshalled here, not for the expert, but for the benefit of biological and other students and non-specialist doctors. In order to avoid interrupting the text by explanatory matter, it has been necessary to use a moderate number of medical and other technical terms. As, however, those for whom the book is intended will presumably have very different backgrounds, a fairly comprehensive glossary is included (pp. 160–162). It is thus hoped to avoid either irritating medical readers by including unnecessary definitions in the text or confusing the non-medical ones by using terms which are possibly unfamiliar to them.

I wish to thank Professor M. G. P. Stoker, FRS, and Dr R. J. C. Harris, of the Imperial Cancer Research fund, for kindly reading and criticizing the text and for other help.

1
Overgrowth and Cancer

Viruses are concerned in the causation of some malignant tumours in birds, mice and other species. This is a fact, long denied, but now almost universally accepted. Comparative pathology teaches us that the causes of disease are much the same throughout the animal kingdom. It is therefore reasonable to argue that viruses may be involved in at least some human cancers also. There is, however, no convincing evidence of this. Most of our knowledge about fundamental aspects of cancer comes from experiments, particularly those in which cancers have been induced to occur in animals, or have been transplanted from one animal to another; so the most obvious lines of research are, for ethical reasons, barred to us when we seek for the causation of cancer in man. Research in the future is likely to find a way around this difficulty, at least so far as concerns the decision whether viruses are or are not involved in human cancers; this will be discussed in chapter 20.

It is wiser to consider whether viruses are involved in the causation of cancer than to ask whether they are *the cause*. Many infections, particularly those due to viruses, are heavily conditioned. It is not a question of merely bringing host and parasite together: many other factors may come into play, and this is very much the case where oncogenic viruses are concerned. Experience with the mammary tumour virus of mice (see chapter 7) reveals that certain cancers result from the interplay of the factors of heredity, viral infection and hormonal environment. If viruses are generally concerned in human or other cancers, it will probably turn out that they are widely distributed agents, causing cancers only when other conditioning factors operate. These conditioning factors, environmental, chemical or physical, may well be the conspicuous things which attract our attention: the role of the virus may be far less obvious. When we come to try to prevent or treat cancer it may be that the chain of causation can best be broken by attacking the virus; but it may equally well be easier to control one of the other factors.

A difficulty arises in the case of some tumours and leukaemias of mice. Some inbred strains of mice have a high natural incidence of malignant disease, from which an apparently causative virus can be isolated. Injection of this virus into young mice may cause a higher incidence and an earlier development of a condition which would eventually appear in a number of the mice anyway. Is this a causative virus or merely an accelerating factor? Probably the best way to look at it is this: if factors A, B and C are needed before the malignancy appears, a lot of factor A (perhaps the virus) will compensate for comparitive paucity of B and C, and cancer or leukaemia will then appear more often and sooner than would otherwise happen.

At first sight there is a tremendous contrast between a cancer and an infection with a parasitic agent such as a virus. Cancer, as such, is not an infectious disease. The same is apparently true, however, of some highly conditioned virus diseases. Herpes simplex virus, though it usually first invades the body in childhood, manifests itself in later life as crops of blisters appearing as a consequence of a variety of stimuli. Much the same applies to the sporadic appearance of shingles in people who have been infected with chicken-pox earlier in their lives. Examples could be readily multiplied.

Many virus infections cause proliferation of cells: in many instances such cell proliferation appears early after infection and is followed by necrosis. Among the poxviruses, vaccinia causes multiplication of epithelial cells lasting for only a few days before necrosis sets in. The proliferative lesions of fowl-pox last for weeks, and indeed the infection has been known as epithelioma contagiosum. Shope's fibroma virus of rabbits causes proliferation of connective tissues which may persist for months before the tumours regress. Normally, however, all these growths are sooner or later surrounded and infiltrated by inflammatory cells, and their proliferative career comes to an inglorious end. It is commonly concluded that these are inflammatory proliferations but not true new growths. Such a conclusion is at first sight reasonable, but it is increasingly difficult to justify when the facts are examined: for it is very hard to draw the line between such overgrowths and cancer. A fowl-tumour virus can induce malignant change in a cell within a matter of days and the resulting sarcoma can go right ahead and kill the bird within a week or two. This sort of thing is probably exceptional: more often the change in the cell from normality to malignancy proceeds by steps. It has been pointed out [120] that the stages of carcinogenesis may be divided into those of initiation and promotion; not every cell which undergoes neoplastic change proliferates and forms a growth. This may happen only with the aid of favouring local conditions, and there is every reason to believe that not infrequently the change is lethal for the cell concerned. Recent work with transformation of cells in tissue culture has made it even more probable that fully developed malignancy is only attained in stages. Moreover, when a neoplasm does begin to grow, its cells are often seen to be very diverse, not only histologically but in their behaviour, so that a tumour may in one corner of its growth be relatively static or even regressing and elsewhere highly invasive.

A danger arises from too great attention to the tumours which have been passed in series, time after time, and have become practically a part of the laboratory equipment of the oncologist. It has long been recognized that transplantable tumours are very different things from spontaneous ones, especially from the point of view of immunology and therapy. There is less appreciation of the possibility that oncogenic viruses after long propagation in series are no longer the same as their wild progenitors; the effects they produce may be much more uniform.

As will be discussed in chapter 19, there is increasing belief that cancer, even without treatment, is not an inevitably progressive fatal disease. Once a growth has reached such a size that it commands attention, that stage may well have been reached. It is, however, likely that there are earlier changes, not clinically detected, which are reversed by the body's defence mechanisms. Appearance of a visible growth is evidence that the defences have been over-run. In experimental studies of virus tumours in animals, we can see more easily that there are indeed defences against oncogenic viruses, that there is a battle with give-and-take on both sides and that either side may win. When the upshot of the fight is victory for the host and the virus-induced swelling retrogresses, it is said that this was not a true neoplasm: but if it has the characters normally associated with malignancy, if it invades and metastasizes, then it is admitted as a genuine new growth. The distinction can be shown to be artificial by the fact that one and the same virus can produce at times a regressing, at other times a progressing, fatal, growth. It may do different things in hosts of one kind, happening to differ from each other in their powers of resistance; or the different outcome may depend upon the age of the host or upon the animal species to which it belongs. Some examples will be given.

The rabbit papilloma described by Shope [324] (see chapter 13 and plate 17) is transmissible both to its natural host, the cottontail rabbit (*Sylvilagus floridanus*) and to domestic rabbits. In both species it produces warts which at times regress: in tame rabbits progression to a malignant epithelioma is quite frequent, while in cottontails it is rare. On the other hand, the fibroma of cottontails, also described by Shope [323] (see chapter 14), gives rise to growths which normally regress completely. When, however, the virus is given to very young rabbits it may produce disseminated lesions and cause deaths (see also chapter 17). The fibromatous growth produced by the typical strain of virus consists of closely packed spindle-shaped cells. A variant strain of the virus has, however, been described [20, 27]: this causes inflammatory lesions with little or no sign of this cell proliferation. Antigenically it was apparently identical with the original strain.

In fowls infected with the Rous sarcoma virus (plate 3) or other filterable fowl-tumour viruses, the outcome depends upon a number of factors including the age and genetic constitution of the birds and the dose and past history of the virus. These factors may all be such as to ensure rapid appearance and continuous growth of a tumour, and indeed workers with the viruses usually arrange matters so that this happens. When, however, things are less favourable, many tumours regress, or, oddly enough, they may apparently regress completely, only to reappear months later. As with the generality of regressive lesions, one sees accumulation of inflammatory cells surrounding, pressing into and overwhelming the tumour. In contrast, the successful sarcomata invade and overwhelm the tissues near them and often give rise to distant metastatic foci.

So, too, with other virus-induced tumours, and not only in them: the warts induced on the skin of a mouse by tar or other carcinogenic agent may, if the chemical treatment is stopped, halt or regress, yet proceed to malignant change if a promoting agent such as the dye Scharlach R is applied.

Enough has been described to indicate that one cannot logically differentiate between true tumours and other lesions, particularly those induced by viruses, on the grounds that some regress and others do not. Nor can histological or other criteria draw this distinction. No one any longer claims that a growth cannot be a cancer because it has a known continuing cause. It has been suggested and will be further discussed that the early stages of malignant transformation may occur commonly and often be reversible. If this is so, the question of definition of the terms 'tumour', 'growth', 'neoplasm' and 'malignancy' becomes more and more difficult. Moreover there is no doubt that, very rarely perhaps, untreated histologically-verified cancers in man regress spontaneously. Practically, of course, these difficulties do not often concern us. A cancer is something which is evident to us because it has managed to grow out beyond the limits of our unaided defensive powers to restrain it, and it will therefore usually kill unless removed or otherwise dealt with. The difficulty of definition only arises when we begin to look deeply into causes and to perceive what has started the cells on their evil course and what struggles have occurred before they have emerged as a declared cancer.

It is of much interest to look back and see in some sort of perspective the fluctuations in the regard paid by research workers and others to the possible role of viruses in cancer. Borrel [48] began it all in 1903, noting that viruses caused cell proliferation and wondering about their possible role in cancer: he did not, however, produce any concrete evidence. Ellerman and Bang [102], when they described a filterable leukaemia in fowls, excited little interest, for it was not widely recognized at the time that leukaemia was in fact a malignancy of blood-forming organs. Rous' description of a filterable fowl sarcoma in 1911 [295] did, however, excite widespread interest and controversy, as will be described in the next chapter. Yet the interest died down, to be reawakened by the claims of Gye and Barnard in 1925 [153] that the fowl tumours afforded a real clue to the 'cause of cancer'. Work on the fowl tumours continued in Britain during the next few years but few workers in the United States showed any interest. A new impetus was, however, given by Shope's discovery of a filterable fibroma in rabbits [323] and a filterable papilloma [324] especially when the latter was found to progress not infrequently to carcinoma. Then Bittner in 1936 described an 'extrachromosomal factor' concerned in causing carcinoma of the breast in mice. Studies of this continued, as did those of Rous and his co-workers on the rabbit papilloma. On the whole, however, and largely because of a necessary change of interest during the war, viral oncology was in the doldrums for a decade or more. In 1951 Gross reported that a virus was concerned in causing leukaemia in a strain of mice with a high natural incidence of the disease. Many workers tried to repeat his work, at first without success. In the end his claims were confirmed, and furthermore, arising from the investigations, there came to light polyoma virus, an agent capable of producing in mice cancers of various sorts. Soon, other leukaemia viruses were described, and the fifties saw an immense resurgence of interest in the subject especially in America. Before long the subject became transformed. Helper viruses which activated more or less defective fowl tumour viruses were described (see chapter 5) and this discovery increased the range of interest in fowl tumours: most surprisingly, it was found possible to transmit them to mammals of several species. Habel [155] and Sjögren and his colleagues [330] showed that polyoma and some other viruses, when they gave rise to cancer, ceased to be demonstrable as infectious entities, though there was evidence that some sort of the virus persisted in the malignant cells. Study of the malignant transformation of cells in tissue cultures added greatly to the interest.

A word of caution is perhaps needed. The 'viral oncology' of the fifties and sixties has devoted its attention almost wholly to strains of virus which have undergone long adaptation in the laboratory and to tumours produced by viruses in unnatural hosts.

The researches will doubtless give an insight into the etiology of cancer, but naturally-occurring tumours must not be lost sight of. There is also a danger that pre-war discoveries may be forgotten: a number of observations made then were very puzzling and might well be capable of re-interpretation in the light of more recent notions (see chapter 20).

2
The Viruses Involved

Oncogenic viruses, those capable of causing tumours, are of several kinds; they belong, moreover, to widely different families of viruses (see table one). There was long dispute as to whether the entities concerned were viruses at all. The fowl-tumour viruses were classed as 'transmissible mutagens'. The mammary-tumour virus was for many years called a milk-factor or an extrachromosomal agent. Such arguments are past and done with: the oncogenic viruses can now be put in their proper places within the known families of viruses. Most of them cause tumours or leukaemias quite incidentally: those consequences of their activity are of no apparent benefit to the virus at all. The polyoma virus is never known to cause tumours in wild mice, though it is prevalent among them as a common inapparent infection. The rabbit papillomata and other warts are, however, presumably transmitted to other hosts mechanically by means of rubbed-off pieces of wart. When, however, they undergo malignant change, this is irrelevant from the viruses' point of view: there is little or no virus in the cancers as compared with that in the benign warts. The rabbit fibromata are probably insect-transmitted: the growths furnish a supply of virus for a biting insect greater than is to be found in the blood or elsewhere.

Classification of viruses divides them into two main categories, those containing DNA and RNA respectively [26]. Oncogenic viruses in these two groups apparently cause tumours in rather different ways. Those containing RNA multiply at the cell surface and normally persist in the tumours they cause. Most DNA-containing viruses, on the other hand, multiply in the nucleus and they may disappear as complete infectious entities, though there may be ways of re-activating them.

Table I. Oncogenic Viruses

	RNA viruses				DNA viruses				
	Fowl-tumour viruses	Mouse mammary-tumour virus	Rodent leukaemia viruses	Myxoviruses or paramyxoviruses	Adeno-viruses	Papovaviruses	Papovaviruses	Poxviruses	Herpes viruses
Examples	Rous sarcoma Avian leukosis	Bittner virus	Gross } Friend } Mouse leukaemias and rat and guinea pig leukaemias	Squirrel virus	Especially types 12, 18, 31	Rabbit papilloma Other warts	Polyoma SV 40	Shope fibroma Yaba	EBV Marek Lucké
Properties of virus family	Enveloped ? Helical	Enveloped ? Helical	Enveloped ?Helical	Enveloped Helical	Naked Cubical 162 capsomeres	Naked	Cubical 72 capsomeres	Enveloped Complex morphology	Enveloped 252 capsomeres
Site of growth	Cytoplasm	Cytoplasm	Cytoplasm	Cytoplasm	Nucleus	Nucleus	Nucleus	Cytoplasm	Nucleus – then cytoplasm
Hosts in which tumours occur — Naturally	Fowl	Mouse	Mouse Rat Guinea pig	None	? 0	Various mammals (mainly host-specific)	? 0	Cottontail rabbit (Shope) Monkeys (Yaba)	?Man (EBV) Fowls (Marek) Frogs (Lucké)
Hosts in which tumours occur — Experimentally	Other birds and mammals (Rous virus)	—	Other rodents	Hamster	Hamster Mouse	Rarely other closely related hosts	Other rodents Ferrets	Other rabbits, hares (Shope) Other primates (Yaba)	Other amphibia (Lucké)

Other characters used in classifying viruses concern their symmetry and other aspects of architecture and presence or absence of a lipid-containing envelope. Most of the DNA-containing oncogenic viruses have cubical symmetry; that is, their nucleoprotein is contained within a rigid box or capsid made up of a number of protein subunits or capsomeres: usually this has icosahedral form. As shown in table one, the adenoviruses have 252 capsomeres (plates 15, 16), herpes viruses have 162 hollow cylindrical capsomeres (plate 1), while papovaviruses have, according to Klug and Finch, 72, the arrangement of which may be skew (plate 14). It is not possible to describe the symmetry of the poxviruses as either cubical or helical. The nucleoprotein in their inner part or nucleoid is in the form of a triad or S-shaped piece, while there are helical strands in the outer coat composed of protein, not nucleic acid. The herpes viruses, besides the complex of nucleic acid and capsid (the nucleocapsid), have, outside this, a deformable lipid-containing envelope. Viruses which have such an envelope are as a rule inactivated by lipid solvents such as ether and chloroform and by bile salts. This applies to the herpes viruses; but not all the poxviruses, though all have such an envelope, are inactivated by ether. Probably, however, chloroform is effective against all. A special characteristic of the herpes virus family is the production of intranuclear inclusion bodies which at some stage are usually acidophilic (plate 2). Virus growth begins in the nucleus and is completed in the cytoplasm. The adeno- and papovaviruses on the other hand complete their development in the nucleus: only the poxviruses, among those containing DNA, grow only in the cytoplasm.

All the oncogenic RNA-containing viruses have outer envelopes and are ether-sensitive. Myxoviruses and paramyxoviruses have helical symmetry, their protein subunits being packed round the helically arranged nucleic acid: they thus have a helical nucleocapsid. Their outer membranes carry projecting spikes with which are associated haemagglutinins, neuraminidase and specific antigens. Their inner structure is readily made visible by the technique of negative staining for electron microscopy and they are easily broken down so that their nucleocapsid is revealed. The structure of the fowl-tumour and mouse-leukaemia viruses (plate 11), on the other hand, is much less readily determined. Surface spikes on the envelope are certainly present on the mammary-tumour virus: they have been reported also for the other viruses causing tumours or leukosis in birds or rodents, but there are no detailed descriptions. Similarly, a helical core has been described for all these viruses but there remains some doubt as to how close they are in their structure to the classical arrangement seen among myxoviruses.

One virus apparently belonging to the myxovirus or paramyxovirus group has been reported to give rise to transplantable tumours after injection into hamsters. This is a virus isolated from squirrels by Vizoso and his colleagues [365]. Since very little is known about it, it will not be considered further.

Neither picornaviruses nor arboviruses are known to be oncogenic but brief mention must be made of the reoviruses, as these have been recovered from Burkitt's tumour (p. 104) and may conceivably be related to it. They are rather small (70 nm.*) RNA-containing viruses without an outer envelope and probably have ninety-two capsomeres. In contrast to other RNA-viruses, their RNA is double-stranded.

If certain, rather ordinary, viruses of various families can cause tumours, it must be that such tumours come about when there is a particular relationship between the virus and host cell. It has been suggested in the case of the adenoviruses that a greater tendency to cause tumours may be associated with differences in the ratios of the nucleotides in their nucleic acids, as compared with less highly oncogenic serotypes: this matter will be discussed later (p. 69). It has also been pointed out that among the papovaviruses, nearly all of which are actually or potentially oncogenic, the frequency of nearest-neighbour base frequencies in their DNA more closely resembles that of mammalian DNA than does that of other virus groups. It remains to be seen whether these clues will prove to be valuable. It must, however, be stressed that, at this stage in our knowledge, there is no justification for using oncogenic potential as an important taxonomic character: many viruses of several families happen to cause tumours under certain circumstances.

* See glossary, p. 162.

3
Fowl Tumours: Early History

The literature on tumour viruses falls roughly into two periods, before and after the second world war. Comparatively few papers on the subject were published between 1940 and 1950 and only towards the end of the fifties was interest really reawakened. Since then discoveries have been numerous and exciting and many ideas have been aroused by these new facts, so that the whole complexion of the subject has changed. An unfortunate consequence is that many workers are unaware of what was accomplished in the pre-war period. In fact, some facts then brought to light were hard to explain at the time, and still are. It therefore seems worth while to mention briefly some of the earlier work.

As mentioned in chapter 1, the first malignant condition known to be caused by a virus was the fowl leukaemia described by Ellerman and Bang in 1908 [102]. Much more impact, however, was made by Peyton Rous's discovery of a filterable fowl sarcoma [295]. This spindle-celled tumour (plates 3, 4) appeared in the breast of a Plymouth rock hen. Rous successfully transplanted it to one of two birds, close blood relations of the original bird; it failed to take in six Plymouth rocks from another source. It was carried for several passes in these 'special' Plymouth rocks and at the fourth passage it infected two of six other fowls. Subsequently it steadily increased in transplantability and malignancy, coming to cause numerous metastases, and it soon went equally well in chickens of any breed. Material from the fourth passage was filtered through paper thought likely to hold back intact cells, and when this gave rise to a tumour, stricter filtration was carried out and it was established that the sarcomata were caused by a filterable agent.

This discovery ran counter to all preconceived ideas of orthodox pathologists, and controversy immediately began. On the one hand it was maintained that Rous' tumour was not a true tumour but more like a granuloma, on the other hand it was urged, and not least by Rous' colleague J. B. Murphy, that the filterable agent was something other than a virus; Claude and Murphy suggested the term 'transmissible mutagen' [64].

Rous himself demolished the argument that the growth was not a sarcoma, showing that in all respects save that it had a filterable cause, it behaved like non-filterable growths in mammals. The metastases were apparently the result of transport of malignant cells, not due to infections of distant tissues by the virus. Growths could be seen breaking into blood-vessels and strands of malignant growth could be seen within blood-vessels. It was shown that immunity in fowls was of two kinds, that directed against the virus and that against the malignant cells [296]. The virus survived desiccation or ultra-violet irradiation as the tumour cells did not: some birds were resistant to dried material but not to cell-grafts, while others gave an opposite result. Tumours regressed in a proportion of birds and these had immunity both against virus and cells [303]. Study of the histological responses in birds with regressing tumours showed that these were like those known to occur in regressing mammalian growths; the reaction, largely lymphocytic, was directed against the malignant cells, not against virus [301]. The sarcomata were not spontaneously infectious and, in fact, apart from the successful experiments with filtration and drying, there was nothing at all to indicate that chicken tumour one was any different from any other sarcoma.

Other workers have isolated similar filterable sarcomata and it is likely that several of different origin are under study at the present time. The history of many is unknown and in the course of years derivatives of Rous' No. 1 tumour have come to differ in serological (see p. 29) and other properties. Logically, only those owing their origin to No. 1 tumour should be called Rous sarcomas. It has, however, become the practice to apply Rous' name to any of the spindle-celled tumours under study. In view of doubts as to the parentage of some of them, this course, though illogical, seems inevitable and will be followed in this book.

The original filterable tumour, whether transferred by means of cells or filtrates, begins to show evidence of growth within a few days of inoculation and normally progresses to kill the birds. Inoculations are commonly made into muscles of breast or legs. When filtrates are injected, it is helpful to add a little kieselgühr or other material to the filtrate, as the virus 'takes' better when it has access to damaged tissue.

The character of the growths varies, both as to its naked-eye appearance and its histology [302]. In relatively resistant birds it may appear white and fairly solid: when in the full flush of malignancy it is soft, diffluent, haemorrhagic and full of mucinous material. Filtration is more likely to be successful if rapidly growing tumour tissue is used, and it may fail altogether with slow-growing tumours [152] (see p. 27). Such non-filterable tumours are then, less than ever, to be distinguished from mammalian sarcomata, though they will regain their filterability when passed through susceptible birds.

Rous and his colleagues were soon able to describe other filterable fowl tumours. An osteochondrosarcoma [362] grew more slowly than did the first sarcoma; inoculated birds showed a fair number of regressions and there was little increase in malignancy after a number of passes. A sarcoma of intracanalicular pattern was fissured by blood-sinuses but, after passage, became more like a simple spindle-celled tumour. In contrast to the finding with chicken tumour one, it took as well in birds of an alien breed, Plymouth rocks, as in brown Leghorns in which it was originally found. Subsequent workers who have encountered naturally occurring fowl tumours have not, as a rule, found that adaptation to birds of mixed breeds was very difficult. It was found [303] that immunity to cells and to virus was largely specific: birds immune to one of the three tumours under study were not necessarily resistant to the others.

More than twenty years after Rous' first discovery there was still controversy as to whether the infectious agent was a virus or something else. It was, however, shown [101] to be particulate, of a size comparable with that of other viruses and, indeed, larger than many of them. A number of reasons for considering it as a virus were marshalled [19]. Its viral nature, is, however, so universally accepted nowadays that the controversy has lost most of its interest.

Rous' last paper on the subject for some time was to show with two colleagues [304] that an antiserum capable of neutralizing chicken tumour one filtrates could be prepared in geese. These were repeatedly immunized with tumour tissue and blood of moribund fowls; the sera had to be absorbed with fowl red cells to remove the anti-fowl element in them.

Rous became discouraged after this by his failure to make pathologists realize the importance of his work. He turned to other subjects and did not resume work on cancer until Shope discovered the rabbit papilloma and the cancers developing from them in 1933 and 1934.

Interest in the subject now shifted to Britain. W. E. Gye at the National Institute for Medical Research began to study the fowl tumour agent, originally to fill in time before things were ready for him to start a programme on dog distemper. Though he leant at first to the view that Rous' agent was not a virus, he was soon convinced that such a conclusion was mistaken. He collaborated with J. E. Barnard, who was developing ultra-violet microscopy, and in 1925 they published a paper in the *Lancet* entitled 'New research into the origin of cancer' [153]. This was soon followed by a book (with W. J. Purdy) with the somewhat pretentious title *The cause of cancer* [154]. It was claimed that a virus had been cultivated in a cell-free medium and that this when inoculated along with a 'specific factor', itself inactive, would reproduce the tumour. Suffice it to say that the claims, though exciting much interest at the time, could not be confirmed. Gye did, nevertheless, succeed in reawakening interest in the 'virus theory', exposing the fallacies of current dogma in the field of cancer.

Gye was one of several workers who studied antibodies against the Rous virus. There is now general agreement that a specific neutralizing antibody develops in fowls or can be induced by inoculating mammals and that this is in every way comparable with the antibodies against other viruses.

It was found also that there were cross-reactions between different tumour viruses but that these were not identical, homologous sera being more potent than heterologous ones [15, 18].

Neutralizing activity was also found in sera prepared by immunizing rabbits or goats with material from normal fowls. Most workers found that complement was required for neutralization by such sera. The result was not surprising for there is plentiful evidence that host components are incorporated in the surface structure of avian tumour viruses.

It was later maintained by Rubin [310] that the results were not due to virus neutralization in the ordinary sense, but rather to a cytocidal action of the serum on the cells of the host into which the virus–sera mixture was injected : the effect was on the ability of cells to divide and form a tumour.

Some fowls transmit immunity to their offspring – a fact which accounts for the variable results of tests of virus in young chickens. It has been shown [22] that anti-Rous antibody, like other antibodies, may be transmitted to chicks by way of the yolk. In very young chicks free from antibody, Duran-Reynals [89] found that intravenously injected virus gave rise not to tumours but to a haemorrhagic disease. There were blood-blebs and diffuse haemorrhages in various viscera and in subcutaneous tissues, and death occurred within a few days. Histological study showed rupture of endothelium without evidence of tumour growth. As progressively older birds were used, a change from haemorrhagic disease to tumour formation was seen. Chicks one to three days old showed predominantly haemorrhagic lesions : in older ones there was more and more neoplasia. Fujinami virus led to similar results, but other viruses produced only neoplastic lesions. Similar findings have been reported in rats (see p. 36). Other workers have not always seen the haemorrhagic disease, perhaps because they were working with more resistant birds or less virulent viruses. Duran-Reynals' finding emphasizes the point made in chapter 1 that there is no sharp line of differentiation between neoplastic and non-neoplastic virus diseases.

The malignant diseases of birds from which viruses have been recovered all involve connective or blood-forming tissues, not epithelium. Experimentally, however, it has been possible to produce changes in epithelial cells. Keogh [189] placed Rous tumour virus on the chorio-allantoic membranes of developing eggs and produced foci of proliferation of superficial cells (plate 5). When, however, transfer was made from such lesions to chicks, only typical sarcomata were produced. It was later shown by Carr [54] that the Rous virus and also that of the fowl endothelioma MH2 would produce adenocarcinomata of kidneys in young chicks. These, however, were not transplantable.

4
Fowl Leukaemias

The viruses causing fowl tumours and leukaemias are members of a family of related viruses; they also cause inapparent infections. The term 'leukosis' is a generic one applying to all malignant conditions of the lymphoid system: 'leukaemia' should be used only when there are also increased numbers of white cells in the circulation. Their relationships have been very difficult to disentangle for a number of reasons. Some of the viruses, though they usually cause a particular pathological condition such as sarcoma or myeloblastic leukaemia, may at times give rise to another of the spectrum of diseases associated with members of the complex [125]. Some, such as the much-studied Rous sarcoma or the BA1 A strain of myeloblastosis breed fairly true: their characters have apparently been fixed as a result of many serial passages. With others, the effects of which are less constant, the explanation is not certain. There may be mixtures of viruses, one or other of which may predominate; and indeed it is known that some 'strains' of virus contain more than one agent. Alternatively, those viruses not fixed by prolonged passage may have the potentiality of infecting different kinds of cells with accordingly diverse results. It is probable that most breeds of hens carry viruses of this family. In fact, those who use chick embryos for making vaccines against other viruses such as yellow-fever or influenza have to take great pains to obtain their eggs from flocks free of leukosis. This means that these viruses are normally quite harmless agents, only giving rise to tumours or leukaemias under abnormal circumstances; and fowls are in fact abnormal birds, bred over hundreds of generations for high egg-production and other desired qualities. It is highly improbable that the wild *Gallus*, from which our domestic birds are derived, have anything like the incidence of these malignant conditions.

The spectrum of diseases caused by these viruses includes sarcomas of several histological types, as described in the last chapter, lymphoid leukosis, erythroblastosis or myeloblastosis: these last are malignancies respectively of the systems producing lymphocytes, red blood cells or myelocytes and polymorphonuclear cells. There are also tumours of the kidney and a bone condition called osteopetrosis (see p. 22).

Yet another confusing factor comes in. All the pathological conditions mentioned involve cell proliferation. In the case of lymphoid leukosis the cells involved are lymphocytes and these may be found in large numbers in the liver and other viscera. There is also a condition known as neurolymphomatosis or fowl paralysis: in this, too, there are massive lymphocytic infiltrations, involving particularly nerve trunks, and until recently this has been considered as one of the members of the leukosis complex. Now, however, it has been shown that the causative agent is a quite unrelated virus, belonging to the herpes virus family. The confusion is all the greater because of the recognition of an acute form of the disease affecting particularly the liver and other viscera and therefore peculiarly apt to be confused with lymphoid leukosis. In the interests of clarity it has recently become the practice to call the disease due to a herpes virus 'Marek's disease', after the first describer, and this is seen to exist in a chronic neuro-proliferative and an acute visceral form (see p. 24).

Properties of leukosis viruses

Numerous studies have been reported concerning the morphological, physicochemical and other properties of members of the leukosis complex. The discrepancies, as between the various members, are probably due to differences in technique, and it is safe to describe all these viruses as essentially similar, except in their biological effects. As was mentioned in chapter 1, they are enveloped RNA-containing viruses. Their diameters are between 80 and 120 nm., and the dry weight of a particle of avian myeloblastosis has been estimated at $7 \cdot 5 \times 10^{-10}$ µg. The density is between $1 \cdot 16$ and $1 \cdot 18$, the amount of lipid being probably variable. Presence of this lipid in the outer envelope is associated with sensitivity to inactivation by ether. As virus is released from the cell membrane by budding it takes with it some host components. From examination of thin sections it appears that the inner core, 35 to 45 nm. across, is surrounded by two membranes. Negatively-stained preparations show the presence of knob-like protrusions from the outer membrane [46, 84] but these are by no means so readily revealed as are the regular spikes of myxovirus; nor has any associated haemagglutinin been demonstrated.

Eckert and his co-workers [97] found evidence of a tubular structure within the core, but this has not been easily broken open as are the cores of myxoviruses and one cannot yet state positively that the core contains a helical nucleocapsid.

The RNA of the virus has an estimated molecular weight of 9.6×10^6 daltons. Though no one doubts that this is an RNA virus, its growth is inhibited by DNA-inhibitors such as halogenated deoxyuridines. It is presumed that functionally-intact DNA within the cell is necessary for virus synthesis. Though fluorescent staining shows that virus is multiplying in the cytoplasm, it is not excluded that events within the nucleus are concerned also. Besides the specific virus proteins, a number of other substances may be detected in the outer coat of the virus. As already mentioned these may include host components; of these Forssman antigen is one. Of particular interest is the presence in particles of avian myeloblastosis of the enzyme adenosine triphosphatase: estimation of the amount of this enzyme has even been suggested as a method of virus titration [246]. It is not significantly present in particles of other leukosis viruses. There is little doubt that the enzyme in the myeloblastosis particles is derived from the myeloblasts which the virus is infecting. The virus can infect also kidney cells and cause a nephroblastoma: virus from such cells is largely free from the enzyme.

Mention was made in chapter 3 of immunological studies of the fowl-tumour viruses: further discussion must be deferred till the question of helper viruses has been considered in the following chapter.

We must now turn to other aspects of the viruses causing the different kinds of leukosis, not forgetting their clinical aspects and their importance to the poultry industry. Altogether they represent the most serious and the most intractable diseases affecting fowls.

The annual loss to the poultry industry in Britain has been estimated to be as high as 7–8 million pounds and in the USA as of
the order of 73 million dollars. These losses probably include
Marek's disease as well as leukosis.

Affected birds show pallor due to anaemia and are listless with
loss of weight and appetite. Diarrhoea may occur in the later
stages, especially in the lymphoid form. All forms are ultimately
fatal. Fowls dying of *lymphoid leukosis* show enlargement of liver
and spleen, but almost any organ may be affected and show massive infiltration with lymphocytes. The lesions may be diffuse or
nodular. The blood may contain abnormal cells but leukaemia is
not a regular feature. At one time it was thought that the disease
was not transmissible experimentally, but Burmester and his colleagues [51] have developed a strain, RPL 12, readily passed in
series; similar strains have been isolated since. The disease mainly
affects fully grown birds.

Erythroblastosis is relatively rare and sporadic though outbreaks
are recorded. There is leukaemia and many immature cells are
present in the blood. There may be severe anaemia: the blood
changes have been fully described [124]. The cells accumulate in
liver, spleen and bone marrow, giving them a cherry-red colour.
There may be as many as 10^{10} virus particles/ml. in the blood. The
virus is readily transmitted experimentally but the disease does
not easily pass as such from chick to chick.

Myeloblastosis is also uncommon naturally. It may occur in a
nodular or a diffuse form. In the former case, tumours may be seen
on the inner surfaces of pelvis, sternum and ribs: they have a
cheesy or chalky consistency. The white blood-count may reach
over 2,000,000/ml. and there may be 10^{12} virus particles/ml.
Liver and spleen are enlarged and the liver may have a fine granu-
lar morocco-leather appearance. Mention has already been made of
the association of adenosine triphosphatase with the virus.

The virus, when grown in cultures of myeloblasts containing
less than 20 per cent fowl serum, showed little of interest [47].
When, however, the serum concentration was raised to 50 per cent,
striking changes appeared. There were many 'grey bodies' within
which virions could be detected. The authors suggested that these
were derived from mitochondria, and that it was in them that virus

synthesis was occurring. A number of clear virus-containing vacuoles were seen and were perhaps produced 'as the substance of the grey body was consumed'.

Osteopetrosis is a non-malignant condition in which there is excessive activity of osteoblasts leading to great thickening of the bones. The causative agent has properties like those of the fowl leukoses and the condition turns up in a proportion of birds inoculated with lymphoid or other forms of leukosis. The bony overgrowth often occurs on one side of a long bone leading to convex curvature on its anterior surface; the medullary canal comes to lie eccentrically. Newly formed bone can be readily crumbled away by the fingers.

Transmission of leukosis

The story of the transmission and general ecology of avian leukosis is a complicated but fascinating one. The basic fact is that adult hens are of two kinds, behaving in different ways [311, 312]. Some are immunologically tolerant to the virus and have viraemia usually throughout their lives. They lay eggs which are infected with the virus. The hatched chickens similarly carry the virus indefinitely, being themselves tolerant. Most of their tissues contain and go on synthesizing virus: yet they grow up happily and normally. Their importance lies in the fact that they regularly shed virus into their environment via the faeces and through the air, and they may thus infect susceptible birds. The immunity of these tolerant birds is, however, by no means complete: the incidence in them of visceral lymphomatosis later in life is definitely higher than in other birds. 'Vertical' transmission of virus through the egg is something dependent only on the status of the hen birds. Viraemic cocks mated to virus-free hens do not cause them to lay infected eggs: this is evidence that the virus dwells in cytoplasm not in nuclei. These viraemic cocks may however transmit infection 'horizontally' by contact.

In the second class of hens there is antibody in the blood but no prolonged viraemia. Such birds have been infected after hatching when immunologically mature, have undergone transient infection with viraemia and have developed antibodies. The eggs they lay contain no virus but antibody is passed on in the yolk, so that the hatched chicks are, for a while, immune. When this immunity passes off, one of two things may happen. They may become infected before they are immunologically mature, and then they will become chronically viraemic shedders, like the first class of hens we have considered. More frequently their passive immunity protects them until their immunity mechanisms have developed: they will then have only transient infections and will become immune hens like their mothers. Once again, the status of the cocks does not affect the issue. And again, immunity in 'immune' hens is not absolute, for some such birds may, later on, develop visceral lymphomatosis. It must be emphasized that it is not all quite as simple as has been described, for there are some switchings from tolerance to immunity in individual cases.

Knowledge of all this is of great importance in relation to the possibility of controlling the diseases in question. It has proved possible to build up flocks of virus-free birds by taking eggs from immune hens and protecting the hatched chicks by rigid quarantine from contact with infected birds. Birds of such flocks are used to provide eggs for vaccine production. In theory it should be possible to free all flocks from these viruses, but the practical application of such theory to the whole poultry industry would involve enormous difficulties.

In the case of myeloblastosis and erythroblastosis, it is clear from the names bestowed on the conditions which are the 'target' cells which the viruses attack. It has become evident from recent work that the corresponding 'target' cells in the case of lymphoid leukosis are in the bursa of Fabricius. The thymus in mammals is known to be intimately concerned in immunity and in the genesis of leukaemia in mice (see p. 52). The bursa of Fabricius is an organ on the dorsal aspect of the cloaca of birds and this carries out some of the functions of the thymus in mammals, particularly antibody formation. In birds, thymectomy in early life does not affect the incidence of leukosis as it may do in mice, but removal of the bursa in birds less than five months old does cause a definite reduction in incidence of leukosis following injection by the RPL 12 virus. Moreover grafts of bursal tissues from normal three-month-old birds into bursectomized chicks restores some susceptibility to this form of malignancy. Dent and his colleagues [80] conclude that

B

the bursa is an important source of malignant cells. Bursectomy does not affect the incidence of erythroblastosis or osteopetrosis.

Marek's disease, as mentioned earlier, was for long considered as one of the manifestations of the leukosis complex, but it is now known to be caused by an entirely unrelated virus. In its most familiar form, chronic Marek's disease causes fowl paralysis, also known as range paralysis or neurolymphomatosis gallinarum. The paralysis commonly begins in birds two to eight months old, usually in a wing or a leg (plate 7). It is associated with inflammatory changes in nerve-trunks leading to great thickening and infiltration with vast numbers of lymphocytes (plate 8): other organs may be affected and at the end the appearances are not unlike those of visceral leukosis. In another form of the disease, the iris is affected. This condition is known as grey eye: the iris loses its colour and there are irregularities in the pupil; finally there is blindness. Neurolymphomatosis has been reported in pheasants, turkeys and quails as well as in domestic fowls. In fowls it was first described in 1907, became very troublesome, but has since decreased.

On the other hand, there has in recent years been a great increase in what is known as acute Marek's disease. This is characterized at first by enlargement and lymphocytic infiltration into liver and other viscera rather than nerves. Lymphoid tumours occur particularly in the gonads and are not unlike those of lymphoid leukosis, but histological studies disclose differences: it is not so easy in acute Marek's disease to maintain that the disease is typically neoplastic. Acute Marek's disease causes high mortality, beginning as early as four to six weeks after hatching. Survivors of the acute disease may go on to develop nerve lesions and paralysis.

Early work on transmissibility is hard to interpret because of the confusion between this disease and leukosis. Once the distinction had been established, it was possible to carry out controlled experiments using birds from flocks of known history. Biggs and Payne [38] showed that the disease could be regularly transmitted to young chicks of a susceptible line; birds fifty days old were more resistant. The disease was shown to be readily contagious, and not only to chicks in direct contact with infected ones but to others in a separate pen in the same room. Infected chicks began to be infectious to others during the incubation period, and infectivity persisted until they died. Oral secretions, not faeces, were infectious: the airborne route seemed to be the important one. It is not known whether infection can be transmitted, as that of leukosis can be, in the egg: most probably it cannot. It was shown that the blood and various organs contained the infectious agent. It proved, however, difficult to establish that there was a virus present in cellfree filtrates. Nevertheless it seemed clear that one was not dealing merely with transplantation of cells, for use of the sex chromosome as a marker revealed that cells from tumours were derived from the host and not the donor birds. Studies of pathogenesis showed that the collections of lymphoid cells in nerves and elsewhere were due to a 'neoplastic-like proliferation'. Demyelination and other changes in nerves were secondary to this proliferation.

In 1967 Churchill and Biggs [62] were successful in cultivating the infectious agents in chicken kidney cells and cytopathic effects were observed in these. Moreover, there appeared in them intranuclear inclusions very similar to those produced by the herpes viruses (plate 2). Addition of inhibitors to the cultures indicated that a DNA-virus was concerned. Finally electron microscopy revealed the presence of particles covered with projections closely resembling those of herpes viruses (plate 1).

There are other examples of transmission to cultures of members of the herpes virus group in the absence of demonstrable filterability. Some of these viruses seem to be closely cell-bound, able to pass to normal cells only by cell-to-cell contact. Thus, chicken-pox material from crusts of human lesions can infect cultures, yet transmission by means of filtrates to fresh cultures is ordinarily impossible. The same is true of the viruses of malignant catarrh of cattle, the virus recovered from Burkitt's tumours (see p. 104) and that associated with kidney tumours in leopard frogs (see p. 99). The need for cell-to-cell transmission may not be absolute: for unknown reasons it has been possible to infect cultures with filtrates of varicella and malignant catarrh, if thyroid tissue is used.

As with the leukoses, breeds of fowls differ in susceptibility to Marek's disease. Genetic experiments are being undertaken with a view to selection of clones of birds relatively resistant to contact infection. Resistance to the acute and chronic forms of the disease runs in parallel but there is no relation to genetic resistance to leukosis, to be described in chapter 5. Recently it has proved possible [63] to immunize chickens against the disease by means of virus attenuated in tissue culture.

5
Defective Avian Tumour Viruses and 'Helpers'

Fowl sarcomata in the course of serial propagation may pass through a phase when they fail to yield active filtrates. Such a happening was first recorded many years ago [152]. Subsequent workers have tried to account for the varying filterability of the virus. It has been maintained that tumours resulting from injecting very small inocula are likely to be non-filterable: also that filtration is more likely to fail if an extract is made from a very slow-growing tumour or from one in an older bird or in one of a relatively resistant strain. All these factors doubtless play a part: yet something much more fundamental has been brought to light. It appears [158] that there exist tumours which are readily transmissible with intact cells but which nevertheless do not release fully infectious virus; the virus in such tumours has been called 'defective'. It is able to maintain the malignant state in the cells which it inhabits but something is lacking in its outer coat, so that it is unable to enter and infect fresh cells. It appears that in many fowls, as described in the last chapter, there exist leukosis viruses, commonly almost wholly avirulent ones: these are able to complement the defective tumour viruses when growing in the same cell. The defective virus is able to incorporate in its surface structure coat protein from the leukosis virus, and fresh cells can thereafter be infected. The leukosis virus is therefore called a helper.

These studies have been made possible by the ability to grow the viruses concerned in monolayers of chicken embryo cells in culture. When fibroblasts are infected with active Rous virus, 'transformation' occurs so that the normally elongated and flattened cells become spherical and refractile, though sometimes they become refractile but remain elongated. They also acquire the power to pile up into layers. Normal cells remain in one layer because of the phenomenon of contact inhibition, when proximity of one cell to another keeps it under restraint (see p. 73). When dilute virus inocula are placed on monolayers of chick fibroblasts, separate foci of proliferating piled-up cells are formed, and these can be counted and so used as a method of quantitatively estimating the amount of virus present (plate 6).

According to timing and other factors, the leukosis virus may either interfere with or activate the tumour virus. The first description of activity of such a virus was by Rubin [313]. He found evidence in some normal birds of presence of a virus which he called RIF (Rous inhibiting factor) because cultures infected with it would not support the multiplication of fowl-tumour virus added subsequently. Later, other viruses were discovered which were called RAV (Rous-associated virus). These and also the original RIF, when inoculated simultaneously with defective virus, would act as helpers. One virologist rudely referred to all these viruses as riff-raff. Presence of one or other can be revealed in Rous-tumour extracts by making passages at limiting dilutions. The RIF or RAV viruses are present to a higher titre than the tumour virus; so one can recover them free from the latter. The fact that many fowl tumours were kept going by the activity of defective viruses was overlooked for many years because the conditions of experiment were such that there were ample opportunities for double infection of cells with viruses of the two kinds.

It is also possible to obtain from some tumours defective Rous virus free from helpers. High dilutions of infected chick embryo cells are plated out, so that only a few foci of transformed cells appear in each dish. The infected cultures are overlaid with agar containing antisera to the helper virus. Some clones of virus recovered after such treatment have proved to contain only defective virus, the cells being capable of indefinite propagation without liberating free virus.

It has been found that strains of Rous sarcoma virus may differ from each other antigenically. The difference may be great so that antiserum against one may be quite impotent against another. In general, this is explained by antigenic differences between helper viruses: for members of the leukosis complex, and thus potential helpers, are diverse antigenically. Differences may be small, though with no two being exactly alike; yet there may be big differences, as between RAV1 and RAV2 strains. The matter has been hard to clarify because some tumour strains, for instance Bryan's high-titre strain, may contain mixtures of three different helpers. When that sort of thing happens cross-neutralization experiments may naturally suggest that two strains are antigenically alike, when in fact they may have but one component in common. When interference experiments are carried out, it is the outer-coat protein which is concerned: accordingly we find, as we should expect, that interference is only fully effective when we are dealing with two antigenically similar viruses.

Thus the helper supplies to a defective virus the properties with which the coat is concerned – the ability to become absorbed to and to penetrate the cell, its behaviour in neutralization tests and the associated events concerned with viral interference. So long as the defective virus and helper continue to be propagated together, these virus properties will remain the same. But the change is not a genetic one, only phenotypic. Take away the helper and the defective virus is just what it was before; it may then be possible to reactivate it by a different helper. The genome of the defective virus can demonstrate its individuality even in the presence of the helper virus. Foci of transformed cells produced in culture may be of several varieties. They may be compact or diffuse according to whether all or only some cells are transformed: the foci may be single or many-layered: the transformed cells may be fusiform or spherical. These are apparently properties determined by the genome of the defective virus and this also must control the replication of the specific viral RNA. Probably also it is concerned with forming the antigen ('COFAL', see p. 37) which is common to all members of the leukosis complex. We thus see that the propagation of one of these complex viruses is a two-stage process. The events just mentioned, probably the early ones in synthesis of new virus, are controlled by the genome of the defective virus, later events concerning surface proteins by the helper. It has been rather surprising to find that in propagated tumours due to helper-free defective virus, some particles, apparently morphologically perfect, can be detected by electron microscopy. This is perhaps easier to explain in view of a recent discovery indicating that defectiveness is only relative, not absolute. Strains apparently quite defective for chickens have been found capable of infecting quail cells. It has been suggested therefore that instead of using the term 'defective' is might be better to call such viruses 'non-producers' [367] or 'leukosis-free Rous virus'. Finally it must be emphasized that defectiveness is a property of only some strains of Rous sarcoma virus, not of all.

Defective Rous viruses (RSV) activated by various helpers are referred to as pseudotypes: we thus have RSV–RAV1, RSV–RAV2 pseudotypes and so on. Different inbred strains of fowls are found to have different susceptibilities to the different pseudotypes: they can in fact be divided into categories on this basis [366]. The genetic susceptibility of fowls is related to the antigenic make-up of the viruses. These, on the basis of their antigenic structure, can be placed in two broad groups A and B, which cross-react only slightly. There are probably other groups, C and D [86], although it is possible that some viruses behaving anomalously may be mixtures. Fowls may be resistant to viruses of the A but susceptible to the B group or *vice versa*: some may be susceptible to both or resistant to both. In genetic experiments the allele for susceptibility seems at times to behave as a dominant, while in the other breeds of fowls it is resistance which is dominant.

Knowledge about defective viruses makes it easier to understand the results of serial transplantation of Rous sarcomata. Transplanted cells give rise to tumours after a shorter latent period than when filtrates are injected: this suggests that the transplanted cells are themselves growing. This can be shown to be the case, for studies of chromosomes allow one to distinguish between male and female cells. When tumour cells from a cock are inoculated into a hen, cells with male chromosomes can be identified. If, however, serial transplantations in hens are carried out, the male cells become less and less frequent and further propagation of the tumour seems likely to be due wholly to infection of the recipients' cells by the virus. As mentioned earlier, transplanted sarcomata may regress in fowls and it is likely that this occurs, at least sometimes, when tumours produced by defective viruses are subjected to a homograft reaction on the part of the host.

6
Fowl Tumours in Other Species

The whole subject of the tumours caused by avian viruses has become much more exciting since the unexpected discovery that they can be transmitted, not only to other birds, but to mammals of various species, including even monkeys. It is interesting historically to note the gradual increase of knowledge concerning the range of species which the fowl-tumour viruses have proved to be able to infect.

Fowl tumours in other birds

The earliest success was reported by Fujinami and Hatano [122]: they transmitted their strain of fowl sarcoma to ducks, birds of a quite unrelated family. This work was later followed up by Gye [150, 151] and Purdy [284].

Gye found that the Fujinami tumour grew well in young ducks of the Khaki Campbell breed but not in Aylesbury ducks. In half-grown ducks tumours reached considerable size but then regressed. In ducklings growth was very rapid and led to death in as little as eight to ten days after injection: the cause of death was obscure, as there were no metastases. Filtrates were also active. Purdy succeeded in propagating the Rous sarcoma also in young Khaki Campbell ducks, but only with tumour mince; subsequent workers, however, have succeeded with filtrates. Des Ligneris [81] was able to produce tumours in guinea-fowls and turkeys by injecting tumour cells, but filtrates were inactive. Some of these tumours regressed but others went on to kill the birds with metastases: indefinite serial propagation in these birds was not achieved. Pheasants were also successfully infected [16, 17], with filtrates as well as with cell suspensions. Serial transfer in young birds was achieved. Some regressions occurred but most birds died with metastases. Cells from other fowl tumours also grew in pheasants. Of particular importance are Duran-Reynals' [90] experiments with ducks. He found, as Purdy had done, that Rous virus injected into young ducks gave rise to tumours; some of these appeared nine to thirty days after injection and were not serially propagable in ducks. On the other hand some of the ducks developed late tumours, 40 to 215 days after the injection, and these behaved quite differently, having characters to be expected of a duck tumour: they could readily be propagated in ducks even with filtrates but were re-adapted with difficulty to grow in fowls. Filtrates commonly failed to infect fowls and serial propagation in fowls was not readily achieved. When it was successful, reconversion to fowl sarcomata occurred more readily from tumours arising in the fowls rather late: in fact the whole sequence was reversed. The duck tumours differed from the original in that they localized particularly in bone and had a different, collagenous, appearance. Later, Duran-Reynals [91] obtained somewhat similar results in turkeys and guinea-fowls. But while he had to use ducks when they were only one day old, he could infect turkeys up to ten weeks old and guinea-fowls up to five weeks. Virus from turkey and guinea-fowl tumours had not lost its affinity for chick tissues as duck-adapted virus had done, but had apparently been modified, having acquired some tendency to produce bone tumours.

Change in the properties of a virus through passage in a strange host is not an unusual phenomenon, yet Duran-Reynals' duck experiments seem sufficiently remarkable to be worth more attention and repetition. There were never any immunological comparisons of the duck and fowl tumours. One wonders whether the late tumours in ducks can have appeared because of 'help' (in the technical sense) by a naturally occurring duck virus. This appears not improbable in view of the finding [195] that young ducks develop 'naturally' an antibody against the duck variant of Rous sarcoma virus. It must be noted that spontaneously occurring filterable duck tumours have not been recorded.

Later, Duran-Reynals recorded that he had succeeded in producing Rous tumours in pigeons, but these yielded no virus and were thus comparable with the tumours in mammals to be described shortly.

Harris and his colleagues [162] found that a strain of Rous virus would not produce progressive tumours in turkeys. They could, however, induce immunological tolerance to chick tissues by injecting chicken blood into turkey embryos or newly hatched birds. Their resistance was thus reduced so that tumours subsequently induced by Rous virus would grow progressively. Svoboda [352, 353] carried out similar experiments using the Prague strain of RSV to which ducks two weeks old or more were naturally resistant. It appeared that the antigen concerned in breaking down the resistance was related to blood-group A substance. After twenty-three passes of Rous virus in young turkeys, Harris found that infectivity for chicks had fallen a thousand-fold while that for turkeys remained high. A single passage in chicks restored high infectivity for them. The changes were thus not as profound as Duran-Reynals had found in ducks.

Fowl tumours in mammals

Despite all these findings there was very great surprise when it was discovered that Rous virus could also infect mammals. Subsequent work in this field has greatly enlarged our knowledge about the virus, and it is at present one of the very active areas of cancer research. First news came from the USSR where Zilber and Kryukova [375] and Svet-Moldavsky [350] produced haemorrhagic cysts, and later, actual sarcomata, by inoculating rats with a strain of virus (Carr-Zilber).

The findings were soon confirmed in Germany by Schmidt-Ruppin [320] and in Czechoslovakia by Klement and Svoboda [202], using different strains of Rous virus. Much of the subsequent findings was reported from Sweden by Ahlström and his co-workers [3, 4, 5, 6, 7]. They were able to infect not only rats but also mice, Syrian and Chinese hamsters, guinea pigs and rabbits. With exceptions to be described, the story is much the same for all these species. It is only a few strains of Rous virus (Carr–Zilber, Prague and Schmidt-Ruppin – hereafter abbreviated at CZ, PR and SR) which regularly infect mammals: others rarely if ever do so. It appears that it is the nature of the protein coat determining the pseudotype which decides whether or not mammals can be infected. It is easier to achieve success by injecting tumour mince, perhaps because more virus can be introduced, but filtrates of Rous virus are infectious also. With the exception of Syrian hamsters, only very young mammals can be infected. There is no doubt, quite apart from the activity of filtrates, that the cells of the mammalian hosts are infected: it is not merely a question of survival of fowl cells; cytological studies confirm this. It can also be excluded that any part is played by polyoma which might be dormant in the mammalian hosts.

The tumours induced may go on to kill the hosts and they have in many instances been passed in series by means of cell transplants: passage to other mammalian hosts with filtrates has normally failed. It might, therefore, have been argued that, as with mammalian tumours in general, there is no evidence of a continuing intrinsic cause of the malignant state. It appears, however, that if these tumours are passed back into fowls, these not only develop tumours but reveal once more the presence of infectious Rous virus. It seems impossible to avoid the conclusion that the Rous genome has persisted all the time in the mammalian tumours but for some reason its infectious character has not been expressed. Two instances are on record in which mammalian Rous tumours have liberated infectious virus: a hamster tumour studied by Svoboda and Klement [353] still contained virus after seven serial passages in hamsters; and filtrates of two rat tumours also infected chicks [348].

Presence of viral genome in non-filterable mammalian tumours has been demonstrated in another way: cells of these tumours can be co-cultivated *in vitro* with chick cells. The chick's cells can then be infected and caused to yield infectious virus, as in the *in vivo* experiments. Presumably there is passage of the essential material directly from cell to cell. Matters may be helped by the presence of an inactivated para-influenza virus, Sendai. A product of the Sendai virus causes lysis of parts of surface of cells leading to fusion of adjacent cells and at times production of multinucleated cells. It even permits fusion of cells of two different species – in this instance mammalian and avian cells. Obviously passage of Rous material into chick cells is made easier in this way.

Attempts have been made to induce mammalian cells which are non-yielders of virus to liberate the active agent: this has been done by seeing whether the Moloney mouse-leukaemia virus (see p. 54) would act as a helper: preliminary tests have, however, given only negative results.

Rous tumours in different mammals show a variety of features of interest. In *rats*, the first mammals to be infected, the appearance of sarcomata was often preceded or accompanied by the development of haemorrhagic cysts. These cysts were often multiple and, when in the peritoneal cavity, sometimes attained an enormous size, containing as much as 20 ml. of blood-stained fluid: they always appeared in the neighbourhood of lymph nodes and at times a cystic transformation appeared in the middle of a lymph-node. The cut surface of the sarcomata was 'homogeneous, greyish-white, moist and shiny but not slimy'. They were invasive and metastasized especially to the lungs. Cells were usually spindle-shaped with nuclei either narrow or round and vesicular [6]. Particles, presumably virions, could be seen in first transplants from fowls, not as a rule in transplants from rat to rat. Filtrates were effective, but inoculations of any kind were successful only in rats less than three weeks old. In contrast to the SR strain of virus, tumours produced by the Mill Hill strain grew for only five to ten days in newborn rats, produced no cysts and could not be serially transplanted in rats.

There is no need to report in detail the results obtained in other species. Mice have been rather less readily infected than rats [4, 211]. Newborn guinea pigs, [3] Chinese hamsters [7] and cotton rats have all proved susceptible, and in the case of Syrian hamsters even adult animals [5]. Rabbits seem to be relatively resistant and their tumours have usually regressed after a few weeks, but fatal tumours have resulted from injection into their brains [287]. Dogs reacted much as did rabbits [286]. In the USSR tumours have been produced in tortoises and snakes [351].

It is of particular interest that monkeys from several species have been successfully infected.

Monkeys. Rhesus monkeys were injected with fowl-tumour material of the CZ strain ; eleven of fifteen newborn animals developed tumours. Juveniles seven to thirty-six months old were resistant unless simultaneously injected with steroid immuno-depressants; tumours then appeared, usually within fourteen days, and most proved fatal. Adult rhesus monkeys were quite insusceptible [253]. Oddly enough, most of the inoculated newborn monkeys developed an acute illness within a few days of injection of fowl-tumour material: they showed weakness, dehydration and loss of weight, and many died. Post mortem revealed generalized arteritis, glomerular nephritis and sometimes cerebral atrophy: the cause was not ascertained [254]. No results of injecting control fowl material into monkeys were reported.

Tumours have been produced also in cynomolgus monkeys (*Macacairus*) and in marmosets (*Sanguinus*). In the cynomolgus they regressed [370] but the tumours in five marmosets were all fatal and metastases were seen [78].

Production of tumours in mammals of so many orders, including primates, raises the question of possible carcinogenicity of the Rous virus for man. This is indeed why such care is now taken that chicken material used in making vaccines for use in man does not contain any leukosis virus. One report is on record of injection of Rous virus into a human being in 1939 [55]. The virus strain was probably related to one which later infected newborn monkeys. However, no tumour had arisen after more than twenty years.

Immunological aspects

Hamsters bearing Rous sarcomata develop in their sera complement-fixing antibodies against an antigen which turns out to be common to the members of the leukosis complex: it is called COFAL (complement-fixation avian leukosis) and is presumably an internal component of these viruses. Complement-fixing antibodies of the same nature appear in rabbits immunized by injection of avian myeloblastosis virus treated with sodium lauryl sulphate. It has been found that mice with Rous fibrosarcomata may or may not develop CF antibodies. With those which do, and only with those, transplantation of the mouse tumours back into fowls gives rise to fowl sarcomata: only one exception was recorded [49]. These fowl sarcomata are usually filterable. At times Rous tumours in hamsters fail to produce tumours in chicks. Such chicks are found to be free of leukosis (helper) virus: when leukosis virus is present the hamster tumours do produce fowl tumours, and filterable ones at that [317].

There will be discussion in chapters 12 and 19 of transplantation antigens: these are antigens not constituting part of the virus genome but concerned in the rejection of transplanted tumours or other cells. Such substances are of course important not only in cancer research but in all work involving tissue or organ transplantation. Several workers [49, 183, 184] have shown that such antigens can be demonstrated in Rous tumours in mice. Mice were rendered resistant to transplantation in one or other of two ways. Syngeneic mice are essentially identical genetically and able to accept transplants from similar mice: such mice were repeatedly immunized with mouse tumours rendered non-transplantable by ultra-violet irradiation. To consolidate their immunity they were given living tumour cells intradermally and the resulting small tumours were ligated so that they fell off: this procedure was repeated a second time. With allogeneic (genetically different or histo-incompatible) mice, it was not necessary to irradiate the injected tumour cells as these would not give rise to progressive tumours anyway. The injection of tumours was repeated three to five times and sometimes the ligation procedure was used also. Mice rendered resistant in either of these ways to tumours induced by one strain of Rous virus were equally resistant to others: in other words the transplantation antigen is something common to all these tumours. There was, however, no correlation between resistance to transplants and presence of complement-fixing antigen, nor with ability to give rise to tumours in fowls.

A confusing discovery is that the COFAL antigen, besides being a constituent of leukosis virus, appears to be present also in tissues of normal, apparently virus-free, fowls of a particular inbred line [83, 276]. The significance of this finding is still not clear. The COFAL test seems to be useful nevertheless in the detection of leukosis viruses [123].

7
Breast Cancer in Mice

In 1936 there was still no general acceptance of the fact that a virus could really cause cancers. It was therefore somewhat of a shock to diehard pathologists when John Bittner produced evidence that a filterable agent was concerned in causing mammary cancers in mice: for breast cancers in women were regarded as the most typical of typical tumours (plates 9, 10).

In 1933 workers at the Roscoe B. Jackson memorial laboratory in Maine reported that in inbred strains of mice, varying in their liability to breast cancer, incidence in the offspring appeared to depend on the ancestry of the mother, not the father. They wrote of an extrachromosomal factor. Then Bittner [39] showed that this factor was transmitted through the milk. In foster-nursing experiments, mice of a low-cancer strain, when suckled by a mother of a high-cancer strain, had a high incidence of breast cancer like that of their foster-mother. Moreover, the agent was commonly passed on again through the milk to subsequent generations. Conversely, potentially high-cancer babies would be relatively free from breast tumours if taken from their mother immediately after birth and suckled by a low-cancer mother. The filterable agent was for years called by Bittner and others 'extra-chromosomal agent', 'milk factor' – anything but a virus; but evidence that it is a perfectly good virus is now conclusive and it is generally known as the mammary-tumour virus or MTV.

The literature about the virus is enormous, for its activities are subject to many influences and are hard to disentangle; a recent review [43] lists over 450 papers, 39 of them being by Bittner himself. Most of the papers make very hard reading, for results are different in various inbred strains of mice and authors have to state repeatedly what mice they were using, whether C3H,

DBA, C57, BALB and so on. Consequently every page of these articles is covered with the letters and figures denoting these strains, until one seems to be looking at a crossword puzzle in code. This chapter will for the most part omit references to the designation of mouse strains; the reader can, if he so desires, follow matters up with the aid of the bibliography.

Progress has been slowed up by many factors. Baby mice infected with the virus may not develop cancers for one or two years: the latent period is always long. Then, the quantitative experiments have been difficult because dilute inocula may give more tumours than those more concentrated. Moreover results of various workers have often contradicted each other. As D. H. Moore [249] writes: ' ... remarkably little has been learned about the nature of this agent. For almost every claim about its properties, there exists a counter-claim.' An important feature brought out by Bittner was that development of breast cancer in mice was dependent on three factors – the genetic make-up of the mice, presence of the virus and activity of hormones. If two only were present, there would probably be no cancer: on the other hand an excess of one factor could to some extent make up for poverty of the other two. These statements need modification in one respect: there are some breast cancers in mice with which apparently the MTV has nothing at all to do.

Mention has been made of the very different incidence of breast cancer in mice of different genetic make-up. There have been many studies of the role of genetics, and numerous genes may be involved. These may affect the propagation and transmission of MTV, the susceptibility of the mammary tissue to change as a result of virus attack or the hormonal milieu. If virus is introduced into mice of a relatively resistant strain, it may not be wholly inactive, but may only give rise to a low incidence of cancers. In subsequent generations in resistant mice these will be even fewer, until finally the activity of virus has been wholly extinguished.

The effect of hormones is seen by the fact that breeding females have more cancers or develop them earlier than do virgins. Forced breeding in particular increases tumour incidence: this means that newborn young are taken from their mother and she is at once mated again and so on, so that she has litters in rapid succession.

Once tumours appear they can be propagated in virgins or males and are thus hormone-independent. A few have been described which are dependent: they grow well during a pregnancy, regress when this hormonal stimulation is over and grow again in the next pregnancy, till finally they go ahead independently of the activity of hormones [119]. Male mice do not normally develop breast cancer but may do so if injected with oestrogens [212].

Baby mice may be infected not only through their mother's milk but by parenteral injection by almost any route. Adult mice may also be infected if very large doses are given. In babies virus diluted $1:10^4$ may infect: the greater activity sometimes seen from giving dilute inocula may be accounted for by the presence of inhibitors, which are only effective at lower dilutions. There is evidence that, rather infrequently, infection may be transmitted from a male parent: probably he first infects the mother, who passes virus on in her milk.

In infected mice, virus is present in many different tissues, though its pathogenic effects are seen only in the mamma. It is in the lactating mamma that highest titres of virus are found: there is more here than in the tumours themselves. The mammary tissue is, however, not apparently infected early on: nor can it be essentially *the* 'target organ', for infection can be established in mammectomized mice.

Virus is also present in the blood and a puzzling feature is here encountered, for such virus seems to have different properties from that in tissues. It appears to be more specific, being only transmissible to mice of the same genotype. Further, it is less readily sedimented and activity is not apparently associated with the same (B) particles as in the case of virus in tissues (see p. 48). It is associated with red, not white, blood cells and may [257] represent a particular developmental phase. Virus does not appear to be excreted in urine or faeces.

The action of the virus on mouse mamma is to produce numbers of hyperplastic nodules: these may be regarded as pre-neoplastic lesions, as it is mainly from them that the actual cancers arise. Like the cancers, the nodules are dependent on hormones for their appearance and maintenance. Not all the nodules are alike; they differ in morphology, secretory activity and aptitude to become malignant. They are well-developed five months after the injection of MTV into baby mice: their appearance can then be used in the assay of the virus and so the observer does not have to wait for answers to questions for the one or two years which must elapse before cancers appear.

Strains of MTV are known, varying in a number of properties, in their tumorigenic potential, affinity for different mouse strains or in the character of the tumours produced. In fact there appears to exist a family of closely related viruses. There are no reports, however, of antigenic differences between these virus strains. Of particular interest is the discovery of a relatively avirulent virus, the nodule-inducing virus [279]: this gives rise, as MTV does, to hyperplastic nodules, but these rarely go on to form cancer. This virus is less readily transmitted by inoculation but can be passed by implantation of mammary tissue. It does not seem to be transmitted in the milk but to be 'vertically' transmitted at conception. It is antigenically related to MTV [43] and appears to be like it morphologically; it and MTV may be present together. Strains of virus exist intermediate in pathogenic potential between MTV and the nodule-inducing virus. Some such have been found in wild house mice [13]: spontaneous tumours have, however, been very rarely observed in wild mice.

Yet other factors are reported to affect the incidence of tumours, factors such as diet, temperature and over-crowding, though these possibly operate by influencing the mouse's hormones. Thymectomy, as will be shown later (pp. 48 and 65) decreases the incidence of mouse leukaemia and increases the number of tumours produced by the polyoma virus. Most reports state that the incidence of mammary tumours is less delayed in thymectomized mice, though there is a record [170] that once tumours have appeared they develop faster in such mice. Several workers record an interference between MTV and mouse leukaemia viruses, the interference operating in both directions.

Properties of the mammary-tumour virus

The electron microscope has revealed particles of two kinds in tissues of MTV-infected mice – whether in cancers, nodules or apparently normal mammary tissue. Such particles were classified by Bernhard [37] as A or B particles: there is good evidence that the latter represent mature mammary-tumour virus. The B particles are 90–100 nm. in diameter, sometimes larger: they contain one, sometimes more, nucleoids which are often placed eccentrically. There are two or more membranes, the outer one being covered with projections. These according to Moore and Lyons [250] are 9·5 Å. long, and spaced about 0·7 Å. centre to centre: they have a central hole and are attached to the membrane of the particle by a relatively narrow stalk. Forms with tails are seen, but these are probably artefacts. There is evidence that virions are released from the cell by a process of budding. Lyons and Moore [224] reported that nucleoids appeared to contain coiled structures 50 Å. in diameter; these may or may not represent RNA-containing nucleocapsids: they were much narrower than those of typical myxoviruses.

The A particles are smaller and resemble in many ways the nucleoids of the B particles. Bernhard considered them as probably a stage in the development of the virion. There is some rather puzzling evidence that activity may be present in some particles considerably smaller than the B particles (see p. 41). Virus particles are present not only in mammary glands and other organs and in the cancers but also in the hyperplastic pre-cancerous nodules and in the milk. They have also been found in tissues of some mice thought to be free from MTV, but it is likely that those represent virions of a related non-pathogenic virus.

The virus contains RNA and has many properties in common with myxoviruses. It contains as much as 26–31 per cent of lipid in its dry weight but such rather unsatisfactory evidence as there is suggests that activity is not necessarily destroyed by lipid-solvents.

Cultivation of MTV

The virus can be cultivated in organ cultures or conventional tissue cultures of mouse mammary tissues: unfortunately there are no readily visible cytopathic effects. Activity of virus can, however, be shown in subcultures and increased numbers of virions are found. While cultures of virgin mammary tissues only survive for about a year, MTV-infected cultures could be kept going for three years [214]: these cultures did not, however, give rise to tumours. In cultures in embryonic cells of another mouse strain, similar prolonged survival of cultures was seen, and, further, some sarcomas appeared when the cultures were inoculated into mice. It is known that sarcomata may develop at times in MTV-infected mammary tumours transplanted in mice over a long time.

From one strain of mice infected with MTV a substance has been obtained giving a 60–70 per cent incidence of adenocarcinoma of the kidney but no mammary tumours [110]. It remains to be shown whether the kidney tumours are produced by a variant strain of MTV.

Several workers have claimed to have cultivated MTV in eggs or in tissues of other species but such claims have been disputed by others.

Immunological studies

Earlier experiments failed to reveal antibodies against MTV, but it has been shown since that neutralizing and precipitating antibodies can be produced by immunization of mice and rabbits [266]. Adequate controls have shown that these antibodies are specific for the virus, being particularly directed to the coat of the B particle. On the other hand, mice bearing the mammary tumours do not have antibodies in their blood. There is evidence for the presence in tumours of a 'soluble antigen', which may be derived from the coat of the virion.

Numerous attempts have been made to show whether or not there are tumour-associated antigens distinct from those contained in the virion itself. Such experiments have been more difficult than those with the Rous virus (chapter 7, p. 38) or with polyoma and SV 40 (chapter 12) tumours, since one cannot, as with those viruses, obtain virus-induced tumours free from infectious virus. Attempts at immunization have sometimes given evidence of resistance to transplantation, sometimes the reverse. It is agreed that as a rule transplantation of MTV-induced tumours is easier in MTV-infected mice than in others: presumably there is tolerance to the virus in those infected when newborn.

It has been mentioned earlier that various strains of MTV cannot be readily distinguished immunologically: also that the nodule-inducing virus is related serologically to MTV. It seems, however, that these two viruses are not antigenically identical, for mice infected with the nodule virus can, when injected with MTV, respond to an antigen present in the latter alone.

There are suggestions, however, that differences between different MTV tumours may be revealed in cross-transplantation tests [363, 364].

Antibodies to MTV do not cross-react with those against viruses of other groups – with one exception: it is reported [347] that a leukaemia in DBA mice contains an antigen which cross-reacts with one in MTV-infected mammary tissue. Mice infected with MTV were tolerant to transplants of material from this leukaemia, as comparable control mice were not.

8

Leukaemias in Mice

The study of viruses and tumours began, of course, with the finding that some avian leukaemias and sarcomas were due to filterable agents. Then Bittner's work on the mammary-tumour virus gave a stimulus to work in this field. But it was the discovery of filterable mouse leukaemias and the incidental revelation of the polyoma virus which really opened the floodgates and made 'viral oncology' one of the most active fields of cancer research. It began with Ludwik Gross, who was studying the AKR strain of mice in which spontaneous leukaemias were quite common. Dalldorf and Sickles had shown in 1948 [71] that the newborn mouse was susceptible to coxsackie viruses which would not infect older animals. Gross [145] produced leukaemia by injecting newborn mice of a low-leukaemia strain (C3H) with cell-free material from the high-leukaemia AKR strain. The inocula were certainly cell-free: the tumours appeared only after eight to eleven months – much longer than would follow transmission by even a few cells: moreover, the leukaemia cells could thereafter be better propagated in CBA than in AKR mice. For several years other workers had difficulty in reproducing Gross' work and there was great scepticism concerning it. But when care was taken to follow his procedures in all their details, it became apparent that his observations and deductions were perfectly correct: there *was* a mouse leukaemia virus.

Work on mouse leukaemias has always been complicated by the fact that many strains of mice have *some* tendency to develop leukaemia spontaneously. If, therefore, the incidence is low or the leukaemias develop late, the worker must always be in doubt as to whether the resulting disease has actually been caused by what he injected. Some strains of mice are dubbed low-leukaemic, but the label may be less justified if the mice are observed for two years instead of one.

Since then, numerous strains of mouse leukaemia virus have been described – already at least twenty by 1962. The astonishing thing is that, apart from Gross' virus, none of them has yet been proved to be the cause of a naturally occurring leukaemia. So far as we know, they are, in nature, perfectly harmless viruses. Nearly all of them have been recovered from propagated mouse tumours and we must assume that they are not the causative agents of those tumours but merely passengers. There is ample evidence that viruses of several sorts, not necessarily oncogenic ones, find in tumours a milieu in which they can grow indefinitely. When such tumours are propagated in series by transplantation, any passenger virus can grow too, and may be quantitatively exalted to a point where it acquires a pathogenicity by no means natural to it. We saw in chapter 6 that there may be tumours caused by viruses, in which no infectious virus can be found; and further examples will appear in later chapters. Here we have the opposite situation, in which tumours readily yield viruses, yet these have nothing to do with causing those tumours. The leukaemic viruses which turn up under these conditions do, however, cause malignant changes of other kinds.

They appear to represent a family of viruses, difficult to sort out and classify. Their pathogenic potential was confused for some time because there appeared, in Gross' experiments, not only leukaemias, but solid tumours of various kinds, especially in salivary glands. These, it turned out, were due to a mixture with an entirely different virus, polyoma, belonging to a quite different family (see chapter 10). This complication has subsequently been sorted out and we know which changes are due to which virus.

Still, however, there is discussion as to how many different mouse leukaemia viruses there are. The safest view is that they are members of a single family of viruses related to that causing mammary cancer in mice and more distantly to the typical myxo-viruses. Differences between them concern their affinity for different cells, their antigenic make-up and a number of other points which will become apparent. They bear the names of their discoverers and the most important ones are the viruses named after Gross, Friend, Graffi, Moloney and Rauscher. Sinkovics [329] has divided them into viruses of the thymic group and the splenic group. The Gross, Graffi and Moloney viruses have particular affinity for the thymus and the incidence of the leukaemias they cause is diminished or delayed by thymectomy: this has no effect on the Friend and Rauscher infections, which localize primarily in the spleen. It appears that viruses of the family are very widespread and it may be hard to find stocks of mice from which they are wholly absent. Recently, viruses of the leukaemia group have been recovered in tissue culture from normal mice of eleven different strains [165]. Their presence in normal and even in ostensibly germ-free mice can be revealed by irradiating the animals: a virus can be recovered from the subsequently appearing leukaemias – a matter dealt with more fully in chapter 17. Studies of 'normal' mouse tissues reveal not uncommonly the presence of particles resembling those of mouse leukaemias [60].

Properties of mouse leukaemia viruses

There have been numerous studies of the properties of the viruses mentioned above [44, 328]. It will be assumed that recorded differences are concerned with differences in technique and that it is safe to consider the viruses as all being alike in their morphology and other fundamental properties.

Mature particles have a dense nucleoid 45–50 nm. in diameter within a thin inner membrane and a thick outer envelope: the diameter of the whole particle is about 100 nm. This is what Bernhard [37] describes as a C particle; it differs from the B particle of the mammary virus in that the nucleoid is larger and not eccentric as it usually is with MTV (plate 11). One can also find in many preparations smaller A particles similar to the A particles of MTV. Several workers have described and figured striking-looking forms with long tails. Most people now believe that they are artefacts, only observel in hypertonic media. De Harven and Friend [76] have described how to obtain preparations in which no tails can be seen. There is dispute as to whether surface projections like those of MTV can be seen: if present they are certainly harder to demonstrate. There was one report that a herpes-like particle with regular capsomeres could be revealed by treating preparations with snake venom; it was later shown, however, that the herpes-like bodies were present in the snake venom itself!

The virus core contains single-stranded RNA with a molecular weight of 10×10^6 [126]: there is some inconclusive evidence as to its arrangement in a helical form, possibly as a nucleocapsid. The outer membranes contain lipid and the viruses are accordingly ether-sensitive: the lipids were studied by Johnson and Mora [182]. At least some preparations have adenosine triphosphatase activity, as has that of avain myeloblastosis. Like other enveloped RNA-containing viruses, these are relatively heat-labile: 20–30 minutes at 56°C. inactivates. Though they are RNA viruses, inhibitors of DNA interfere with their growth just as in the case of fowl leukosis viruses (see p. 20): evidently their multiplication depends on presence of functioning DNA.

Antigenic characters

Neutralizing antibodies have been prepared by immunizing rabbits, but the data obtained have not been quantitative and more information has been obtained by the use of complement-fixation, gel diffusion, immunofluorescence and cytotoxic tests. Workers have not all reached the same conclusions as to relationships, but it is fair to say that many cross-reactions can be detected yet all the viruses have some specificity. Sera from rats bearing lymphosarcomas produced with Rauscher virus contain complement-fixing antibodies reacting pretty well with all the mouse leukaemia viruses. These must contain a common antigen similar to that reacting in the COFAL test among the fowl viruses (see p. 37): it differs, however, in that it is probably a surface rather than an internal antigen. There seems no doubt that the Friend, Rauscher and Moloney viruses are rather closely related to each other and much more distantly to the Gross virus. Old and Boyse [266] state that five antigens are recognizable. One is characteristic of the Gross virus and leukaemias in other mice with spontaneously high incidence (G antigen). Another (FMR) is common to the Friend, Moloney and Rauscher agents. A third is shared by some leukaemia viruses and the mammary-tumour (chapter 7, p. 45). Two others are recognizable in other leukaemias. Mice do appear to develop some antibodies to the viruses infecting them except when they are congenitally infected and immunological tolerance operates. Schäfer and Eckert [318] found that a complement-fixation test could be used with the Friend and Rauscher viruses and that the active sera appeared to detect the specific antigen also in most, but not all, permanently propagable tissue-culture lines: these may well have been carrying avirulent strains.

Tissue cultures

All the strains mentioned have been cultivated *in vitro*. Tissues of infected mouse spleens or thymuses have continued to yield virus into the medium but cytopathic effects have usually not been seen. Similar results have been obtained when the viruses have been added to normal tissues, most frequently fibroblasts from mouse embryos or spleens. These results have not been achieved at all easily, and serial propagation in culture has often failed, perhaps because of inhibitors present in the inocula. Recently it has proved possible to infect continuous lines of cells with several viruses, achieving a 'steady state' with virus being continuously liberated in the absence of obvious cytopathic effects. Most workers have failed to demonstrate transformation of cells in culture such as has been seen with fowl tumour and other viruses. It is possible that when this does occur it is accounted for by the presence of mouse sarcoma virus (see p. 55). Some viruses after long cultivation have lost much of their ability to produce leukaemia although, as judged by electron microscopy, virus particles are still being freely produced.

Pathogenesis

In most infections due to these viruses, there is no great excess of circulating white blood cells. It might, therefore, be preferable to consider the commonest form of the infection as a disseminated lymphomatosis rather than leukaemia. The picture of lymphosarcoma is seen in the thymus, spleen and lymph-nodes, with emphasis on the thymus and spleen respectively in the two pathological varieties of disease mentioned earlier. A leukaemia blood picture and invasion of non-haemopoietic organs occur in the later stages. Affected organs show sheets of tightly packed neoplastic lymphoid cells: mitoses and pyknotic cells are numerous. At an early stage of an infection there is hyperplasia of lymphoid cells and these are not at first malignant: subsequently they become independent of the host's control mechanism and become autonomous. There has been considerable discussion as to why leukaemia following inoculation of Gross' virus only appears after many months, in contrast to the rapid action of another oncogenic RNA virus, that of the Rous sarcoma. It has been suggested that the change to malignancy in mice is the last in a series of steps taking place over a period.

The various viruses have in general affinities for particular cells and particular organs: but the differences are not absolute. As was seen with the fowl tumour viruses, occasional hosts may develop malignancies of cells of a different type from usual. When mice are spared from early death from lymphomatosis as a result of thymectomy, they may later develop a myelocytic leukaemia: this could be because, without the thymectomy, they would not have lived long enough to suffer from that form of disease. The myeloid leukaemias could be transplanted as such for several generations, but filtrates usually gave rise to lymphoid leukaemia [147].

The evidence is good that a number of these viruses are transmitted 'vertically' from mother to offspring: Gross' virus has been obtained from embryos. There is no evidence for 'horizontal' transmission to contacts: no virus has been recovered from faeces, urine or saliva. Nor is there evidence for transmission by the father. Some workers have failed to demonstrate transmission by the mother's milk, but Law [215] could readily show this with the Moloney virus. More resistant strains of mice may fail to pass the virus 'vertically' though they can themselves be infected by injection when newborn. Most of the well-studied leukaemia agents have proved to be transmissible to young rats and, at least in the case of Moloney's virus, to newborn hamsters [244].

Special features of individual virus strains can now be reviewed, and first comes *Gross'* virus. The high-leukaemia strain AKR has an incidence of 85–95 per cent of leukaemia, the disease beginning in six to seven months: most mice are dead by fourteen months of age [147]. When Gross first transmitted the disease from AKR to baby C3H mice the incidence was not very high and the latent period long. Later he was able to develop his A strain by serial passage in baby mice, selecting for each passage material from the mice which developed leukaemia first. This gave much more consistent results, and would infect not only newborn but mice up to ten days old and, less regularly, young adults. After twenty-seven cell-free passages it produced leukaemia in 99 per cent of susceptible mice after less than three months. It has been suggested that the AKR mice are more sensitive to the virus than are other strains because the large cells in the thymus which are, in part, the target for the virus persist longer than they do in other mouse strains. It is however no longer thought that the virus multiplies only in thymic cells: possibly [239] the thymus provides the best environment in which lymphocytes can develop into autonomous leukaemia cells. It should be mentioned that the relative freedom from leukaemia which follows thymectomy is no longer seen when such mice receive homografts of thymus from a mouse of a compatible sort.

An interesting fact is that mice of the AKR strain, which are apt to get leukaemia anyway, develop it sooner if they are injected with Gross' virus. This may be because the date of onset depends on the build-up of virus to a certain level and addition of more virus helps this. Or possibly, as suggested earlier (p. 2) when several factors are concerned in producing an effect, an excess of one may compensate for paucity of another. The interesting question is, however, raised: how far can an accelerating agent be regarded as causative?

Friend's virus [121] has provided a number of puzzles. It was originally obtained apparently from the spleen of a mouse with a transplantable carcinoma, but it is possible that the manipulations activated a virus already present in the inoculated mice. Mice inoculated with the virus soon develop great enlargement of liver and spleen, especially the latter: even seven days after inoculation the spleens are larger than normal and a method of titrating the virus has been based on increases in spleen weight. Nevertheless the course of the disease normally runs for two or three months, though many mice die earlier from rupture of the spleen. Lymphnodes also are enlarged and immature cells massively infiltrate

marrow, spleen and liver. Splenectomy does not significantly pro-
long life, though the first histological changes are found in spleens.
Passage from mouse to mouse goes equally well with cells or filtrates and several types of experiment yield evidence that transplantation of cells is not involved, only infection by the virus of
host cells. Thus neutralization tests can perfectly well be
carried out using cell suspensions instead of filtrates, passive transfer of immunity with antiserum is possible and vaccination with
formalinized virus will protect many mice. Such tests are made
easier by the fact that there is no need to use newborn mice of an
inbred strain: one can infect adult mice of an ordinary stock of
Swiss mice. Such a result would not be expected if one were dealing with a malignant condition, propagable by cell transplantation
in randomly bred hosts.

Pope [280] has described an avirulent Friend-like virus in wild
mice in Queensland. It was serologically related to Friend virus
but produced only chronic infection with lymphoid hyperplasia.

The typical proliferating cell in Friend's leukaemia is of
medium size, often with two or three nucleoli and often having a
kidney-shaped nucleus. Chamorro and colleagues [57] call it 'the
Friend cell'. It and giant cells in the bone marrow seem to be the
chief producers of virus. The virus seems to be multipotential,
stimulating also erythroid cells and reticulum cells. The blood may
contain primitive cells up to 300,000/cu. mm. Several facts suggest that it may represent a mixture of viruses. It has been
suggested [237] that the disease is a leukaemia of reticulum-cell
type combined with erythroblastosis. Mirand and Grace [240]
found that inoculated mice would pass the disease to their offspring, mainly in the milk, but that the young so affected showed
the reticular cell disease, but anaemia rather than erythrocytosis.
Similarly, Dawson and colleagues [73] found that by passing the
virus through rats they could reproduce lymphatic leukaemia but
not the typical Friend disease with erythroblastosis. They were
able to compare the original Friend virus with the rat-passaged
one and found them immunologically alike. The latter, though not
wholly resistant to ether, was more so than typical Friend virus.
No success attended attempts to free Friend virus from the other
agent. Among tentative explanations offered is the intriguing

one that the erythroblastosis-causing virus may be incomplete, requiring the other virus to function as a helper. Mirand and his colleagues [241] describe polycythaemic strains of Friend virus which produce foci of changed cells in the spleen: they, too, suggest that there may be two viruses in Friend leukaemia material, one acting as a helper of the other.

Another agent, which may be related, is described by Kirsten *et al.* [197] as murine erythroblastosis. It was obtained from lymphomas in mice, caused much proliferation of red-cell precursors, but anaemia rather than polycythaemia. It produced malignant lymphomas on passage to baby rats and also erythroblastosis.

Rauscher's virus is very similar to Friend's, producing, like it, splenic enlargement as well as lymphomatosis. Gross [148] has suggested that it may be a mixture of his own and Friend's virus. Many studies of its properties have been carried out but these have been reviewed earlier in the chapter.

Moloney's virus [243, 244] produces a straightforward lymphatic leukaemia without the effects on the erythropoietic system of the Friend and Rauscher viruses. However, it is to be grouped immunologically with those two viruses. Klein and Klein [201] used this virus in experiments seeking for evidence of transplantation antigens (see p. 82). Evidence for the presence of these was found, though no cell-lines could be obtained which did not produce free virus. It appears that a novel cellular antigen revealed in these experiments is shared by the Moloney, Friend and Rauscher viruses, while that of the Gross virus is different. Cytotoxic antibodies are probably directed against the same antigen.

Graffi's virus [138] causes a myeloid leukaemia, sometimes referred to as chloroleukaemia from the greenish colour of affected organs. It is related serologically to the Friend, Moloney and Rauscher viruses. Some preparations have been contaminated with Gross' virus.

A number of other strains with more or less differing properties have been described. Filterable leukaemias arising after irradiation are considered in chapter 17.

Solid tumours

Harvey [166] and Moloney [245] independently obtained from rodents inoculated with Moloney's virus producing solid tumours: these agents are referred to in the literature as mouse sarcoma virus (MSV (H) and MSV (M) respectively). MSV (H) produces inflammatory lesions as well as anaplastic sarcomata or angiomata at the site of inoculation in newborn mice, rats and hamsters: also splenomegaly like that caused by the Friend virus. The MSV (M) tumour has been described as a rhabdomyo-sarcoma [245, 277]. These viruses are like the mouse leukaemia viruses morphologically (plate 11) and resemble them in their basic properties. Tumours could be produced [109] in mice of two breeds and their hybrids: regressions occurred in a different percentage in the various mouse strains. Adult mice could also be infected, but regressions were the rule unless resistance was re-duced by X-raying the mice. Law and his colleagues [216] found that thymectomy increased the number of takes, but even so many quite large tumours ultimately regressed. Transplantation of cells was unsuccessful unless the mice were X-rayed or thymectomized. They considered that the tumours were 'atypical granulomas' but probably contained some neoplastic cells.

The MSV (H) virus was reported to be partly neutralized by antisera against Friend and Rauscher viruses. MSV (M) prepara-tions apparently contain also some Moloney virus but attempts to separate it from the MSV were unsuccessful. Nor could the sar-coma virus of MSV (H) be separated from the agent causing splenic enlargement [230]. Possibly, however, it is all the same contaminated with Friend or Rauscher virus [327]. Inoculation of mice with Moloney virus induced resistance to transplantation of MSV (M) tumour cells.

This confusing picture has been at least partly clarified by the results of tissue cultures. The viruses can be cultivated in mouse cells, especially embryonic ones, and produce in them foci of piled-up 'transformed' cells, as the leukaemic viruses in general fail to do. Apparently preparations of MSV (M) consist of a mixture of focus-forming and non-focus-forming particles, the latter being in the majority: they can, however, be induced to form foci in the

C

presence of Moloney or Rauscher viruses [114, 164]. In other words they appear to be defective and to be rescued by leukaemia viruses in somewhat the same way as was described for fowl-tumour viruses in chapter 5. There is, however, a difference: in the mouse system the helper is required in order to produce foci of cell transformation: with the fowl-tumour viruses its effect is to make transformed cells into yielders of infectious virus.

Simons et al. [327] considered that MSV (H) growing in mice was not defective and required no helpers, while O'Connor and Fischinger [263, 264] held that MSV (M) virions were at times competent by themselves and that the competent particles were actually complexes of defective particle plus helper.

The viruses will also infect hamster cells in cultures and in these foci of transformation are more readily produced than in mouse cells. The cells changed by MSV (H) are spindle-shaped and readily release virus into the surrounding medium. Inoculation of such cells into newborn hamsters gives rise to tumours which in turn release MSV. On the other hand it appears that MSV (M) growing in hamster cells is always defective and requires rescue by a leukaemia virus [176].

The competent viruses so produced are of various 'pseudo-types', as with fowl viruses, according to which leukaemia virus is active as rescuer (cf. p. 30). Even though MSV (H) may not be wholly defective, it was found by Bassin et al. [32] that addition to it of Moloney leukaemia virus increased the number of foci of cells transformed in tissue culture. These authors, after passing their virus through newborn hamsters were later able to establish a transplantable sarcoma in adult hamsters. In culture these cells yielded a virus which gave rise to tumours in newborn hamsters but not in mice. If, however, the cells were grown in mixed culture with mouse embryo cells and superinfected with Moloney virus, one then recovered a mouse sarcoma virus infectious for mice. The ability of leukaemia viruses to act as helpers has provided a useful tool for titrating these viruses. Foci of transformed cells can be counted in as short a time as six days: one does not have to wait for weeks or months for the development of leukaemia in inoculated mice.

It has been reported [265] that the Friend leukaemia virus also may at times give rise to solid tumours. From some of the tumours so obtained there has been difficulty in obtaining infectious virus, but it may be 'rescued' with the help of Moloney virus [114].

A filterable osteosarcoma of mice has also been described [116, 188]. Filtrates injected into mice subcutaneously led to appearance of growths chiefly in the spinal column. Electron microscopy revealed particles similar to those of murine leukaemia viruses.

9

Leukaemias in Other Mammals

Leukaemia has been reported to occur in mammals of many species besides mice and men and others described below: among those mentioned are sea-lions, buffalo, skunks, squirrels, civets, opossums, kangaroos, rats, 'monkeys', deer and elephants [232]. In very few instances has a search been made for a causative virus and one can only guess at whether the etiology is similar for all. It has already been mentioned that murine leukaemia viruses will infect rats and hamsters. A spontaneously occurring filterable leukaemia of rats, has also been recorded [349].

Guinea-pig leukaemia

A spontaneous leukaemia occurring in guinea-pigs [270, 271] could readily be transferred by injecting cells or filtrates into animals of the same strain and also to first-generation crosses of this strain with animals of a resistant strain. It was not necessary to inject only young animals. Evidence of disease appeared in twelve to fifteen days after injecting cells, a few days later after filtrates. All guinea pigs were dead about a week later, often suddenly. It was suggested that the disease more closely resembled chronic lymphatic leukaemia in man than do other experimentally studied leukaemias. Infection was associated with counts of 100,000 to 350,000 white cells/cu.mm. of blood, the cells being primitive lymphoblasts having about twice the diameter of mature lymphocytes. There was infiltration of almost all organs with these cells. One hundred serial passages have been carried out, and infection has been achieved by giving leukaemia cells by mouth as well as by injection.

Electron microscopy of cells in tissues has revealed particles 80–90 nm. in diameter, resembling immature particles of the C type described for murine leukaemias: they were seen budding into cisternae of the endoplasmic reticulum. In intercellular spaces and in pellets obtained by centrifuging blood, mature C particles 90–100 nm. across were seen. The particles were said to be rather smaller than those of the murine viruses and in the immature form the intermediate layer in the virion was not as electron-dense. It is safe to assume that the particles seen were indeed those of a virus, and it is probable that they were the causative agents of the cavian leukaemia.

Leukaemia in cats

Leukaemia is one of the commonest malignant conditions in cats, comprising about 15 per cent of the total. Jarrett [180, 181] describes three forms – multicentric, thymic and alimentary, named according to the chief sites of lymphatic enlargement. Of forty-eight natural cases, numbers in the three categories were fourteen, five and twenty-two, respectively: a few did not fall into any of these groups. The diseases are perhaps best called generalized lymphomatosis, as there is often no excess of white cells in the blood. Material from a cat with the thymic form was used to make a cell-free suspension and some of this was injected into four kittens of a litter. All had developed enlarged lymph nodes six months later and the animals died or had to be destroyed nine to eighteen months after inoculation. All had lymphosarcomata of the multicentric type: there was enlargement of many lymph-nodes and of the spleen. The chief malignant cell type had a large nucleus filling most of the cell and there was at times a foamy area in its cytoplasm: this contained many virus-like particles about 100 nm. across. A dense nucleoid with two surrounding membranes was 60 nm. in diameter and the virions in fact closely resembled those of the murine leukaemias. Similar particles have been seen in the organs of spontaneous leukaemias in cats, and also in cultures of affected mesenteric lymph-nodes. A second passage was made from one of the originally infected kittens and leukaemia has been produced with material from a further field case. It has proved possible to obtain a close association between a mouse sarcoma virus and that of cat leukosis. The complex virus so obtained could be cultivated in cat but not mouse cells: so presumably it had obtained an outer feline coat. Later addition of mouse leukaemia virus restored the ability to grow in mouse cells [118]. It has also been reported that there is a common antigen, shared by the feline and murine viruses [128].

The 'cell-free material' used in some of these experiments was obtained by centrifugation, not filtration. It was thought unlikely, however, that any cells had survived freezing, thawing, grinding and centrifugation, particularly as no tumours appeared near the sites of subcutaneous inoculation. No success followed attempts to produce transformation or other changes in cultivated cat tissues of various kinds.

Leukaemia in dogs

Though leukaemia in dogs is also common, especially in boxers and cocker spaniels, no cell-free transmissions are reported. There is, however, a report of finding C-type particles in lymphatic tissues of two dogs with reticular-cell leukaemia [59].

Bovine leukaemia

In some European countries leukaemia in cattle is sufficiently common to be of considerable economic importance. Evidence that a virus is concerned is at present only suggestive and many attempts at transmission with filtrates have been unsuccessful [96]. Two different conditions may be involved. One, a sporadic form of the disease, is widely distributed and affects mainly calves. The other form, affecting older animals, occurs apparently as a late development of a disease in which there is a benign lymphocytosis: there is, however, argument concerning the relationship between this and leukaemia. It appears definite, however, that the leukaemia of older beasts occurs in clusters, particularly in families, and there are suggestions that it may be transmitted by the bull. In Scandinavia it has a high incidence in certain areas, in contrast to what is found with the form occurring in calves. There has been a 50 per cent reduction in incidence in Denmark following slaughter, quarantine and disinfection: one cannot, however, be certain what part these measures played. Several reports indicate that the disease has appeared elsewhere following the introduction of animals from Denmark or other badly affected country. Leukaemia has been reported as occurring in offspring of a leukaemic cow removed by Caesarian section.

Dutcher and his colleagues [95] have described C-type particles like those of murine leukaemia in cultivated tissues from cattle with lymphosarcoma and have also found them in the milk: their diameter was about 100 nm. Cultures from 75 per cent of leukaemic cattle show a resistance to infection with vesicular stomatitis viruses and this resistance has the character associated with interferon production. This production of interferon is what is commonly found in cultures chronically infected with a virus. However, the authors were not successful in conferring on normal bovine cells this capacity for interferon production, using preparations of cow's milk containing supposed bovine-leukaemia virions.

Human leukaemia

Some forms of leukaemia in man closely resemble some of those in other species and the opinion has been expressed that if any human malignancy turns out to have a viral cause, it will be leukaemia. At present, however, the evidence is slender. An agent has been recovered from human leukaemias which will, it is claimed, accelerate the appearance of leukaemia in mice. Several observers have described 'clusters' of leukaemic children and have obviously felt it possible that an infectious agent was concerned. In Newquay in Cornwall seventeen cases occurred within a short period within a radius of one mile [66]. In a school in a Chicago suburb six cases of leukaemia turned up within a year. Clearly, however, clusters could occur by chance or as a result of some common factor other than an infectious agent.

Again, several workers have described virus-like bodies in preparations of human leukaemic blood or bone-marrow, or in the cultures of these. The particles are said to resemble the murine leukaemia viruses. Others have failed to find such particles or have found them equally in controls. Particles resembling herpes viruses have also been found in human leukaemias: these are likely for the most part to be the EB virus to be discussed in chapter 16. One could point out, if one were an advocate of the virus theory of human leukaemia, that virus particles may be equally hard to find in some leukaemias of mice: while if one were an advocate on the other side, one could stress the occurrence in experimental animal tumours of viruses which were mere passengers. Some of the agents recovered from human material, for example that of Negroni [258] were thought at first to be viruses but were later shown to be mycoplasmas. Negroni's was *M. pulmonis*, an organism frequently found in rats. The mycoplasmas have in fact bedevilled a lot of work in the virus field, for they may be carried undetected in tissue cultures for an indefinite period and be hard to get rid of.

No conclusion is yet possible as to a possible role of viruses in human leukaemia. Even if experimental transmission in man were possible, a ready answer might not be obtained: the different behaviour of the agents of the leukaemia viruses of mice, guinea pigs, cats and cattle should make that clear.

Tumours in hamsters

It is convenient to mention here two transplantable tumours in golden hamsters. One was a pigmented melanoma which could be transmitted by means of filtrates. It was passed more than fifty times by means of cells inoculated into the anterior chamber of rabbits' eyes. In the course of passage it became amelanotic but later regained its pigmented character. Particles resembling Bernhard's C bodies were seen: they were 80–90 nm. across [108]. In another instance [139, 141] multiple skin tumours contained many papovavirus particles; yet transfer to newborn hamsters gave rise to leukaemias in which C particles, like those associated with other leukaemia viruses, were present [140].

10
Some DNA-Containing Tumour Viruses

A number of DNA-containing viruses can cause cancers, and it will appear that their mode of action is in several respects different from that of the RNA-viruses dealt with up to now. The site of replication of most of them is in the nucleus, and it will be a recurring theme that infectious virus may disappear from the tumours caused. Yet something of that virus remains, perhaps closely integrated with the cell [113], and by appropriate means complete virus may at times be 'rescued'.

This chapter will deal with two papovaviruses, polyoma and SV 40, and with the group of adenoviruses: viruses causing warts are the subjects of chapter 13. Those in this chapter have this in common: in their natural hosts they cause wholly inapparent infections or else relatively trivial ones not obviously related to cancer. Their oncogenic potential only becomes apparent under artificial conditions, after transfer to strange hosts, particularly hamsters, or after cultivation or other manipulation in the laboratory.

Polyoma

The polyoma virus first came to light in the course of Gross' experiments on mouse leukaemia [146], as mentioned in chapter 8. When he inoculated filtrates of leukaemia material into newborn mice some of these developed not leukaemia but solid tumours, especially of salivary glands. It was not long before the discovery that these were caused by a virus quite different from that concerned with the leukaemia. This was obtained, free from leukaemia virus, when attempts were made to grow the leukaemia in tissue culture [337]. The tumours caused were of many kinds, adenocarcinomata of parotid glands and kidneys, fibrosarcomata in various places. Pathologists use the suffix -oma to denote tumours of various tissues and organs: so the name 'polyoma' was coined to denote a virus capable of producing tumours of *many* kinds.

Properties of polyoma virus

Polyoma belongs to the papovavirus family (plate 14). Its diameter is about 45 nm., a little less than that of the papilloma viruses which are also included in the papovaviruses. Papova is a tele-scoped form of PApilloma POlyoma, while the VA stands for Vacuolating Agent, another name for SV 40, the next to be considered [235]. The fact that Papova in Russian means the daughter of a priest is an unfortunate coincidence. There is no lipid-containing envelope. There was dispute as to the number of capsomeres, but most workers now accept Klug's view that there are seventy-two [204]; occasional filamentous forms of the virus occur, probably as a result of a fault in the assembly process. Virus particles are found in large numbers in nuclei of affected cells, often regularly packed: larger forms are seen in the cytoplasm. Haemagglutinins are present, and these are not separable from the virions: cells of guinea pigs and other species are agglutinated in the cold [99].

Polyoma virus can be cultivated in embryonic and other cells of mice and other rodents, and destructive effects may be seen. Plaques may develop on monolayers and may be used as a means of assay. This productive type of infection will be contrasted in the next chapter with the events leading to cell transformation and production of tumours. The separated DNA of the virus can also initiate infection.

Natural history of polyoma

Polyoma exists as an endemic inapparent infection not only in laboratory mice but in wild ones too, both in town and country [177]. Its presence can be detected either by isolation of the virus or by finding haemagglutinin-inhibiting antibodies in the sera of the mice. It seems that the virus is not transmitted vertically as leukaemia viruses may be but that it is excreted in the urine:

young mice in a colony are probably mostly infected by exposure to materials contaminated by this. The striking thing is that polyoma tumours are unknown among wild mice. The explanation is not far to seek. The virus normally only causes tumours when very young animals are infected. Moreover, the incubation period is related to the dose of virus – the less virus the longer the incubation period. Infected mothers pass antibodies to their babies through the milk and placenta, and there is very little chance that mice will ingest a lot of virus when very young. If they were infected it would probably be with a very small dose not likely to give rise to a tumour for a very long time: and wild mice don't live very long.

Pellets used to feed laboratory mice may easily come from sources contaminated with polyoma virus from wild mice. By now many stocks of tame mice are certainly infected, and within a laboratory, infection spreads readily. It has thus not unexpectedly happened that cancer-workers have sometimes had a polyoma virus picked up by their mice and have thus been led to erroneous conclusions [307]. Though infection may be transferred in this way, tumours are not caused except in the instance of mice subjected to thymectomy, a procedure which greatly lowers their resistance [216].

Pathological effects

Newborn mice of several but not all strains react to subcutaneous or intraperitoneal injection of virus and in a variety of ways. They may develop carcinomata, most commonly in the salivary glands, or sarcomata of various tissues. The incubation period is usually from three to twelve months. Mice injected when older occasionally develop tumours but only after a very long interval. Polyoma tumours behave like other transplanted tumours in that they will only 'take' in genetically similar mice. As will appear, the tumours are commonly free from infectious virus. Some baby mice instead of developing tumours fail to grow and die if removed from their mothers: or they may show anaemia, conjunctivitis and other effects.

Rats are less susceptible, but may develop kidney sarcomata (plate 13): the fibrosarcomata which can be produced in young rabbits commonly regress [100]. Even young ferrets may develop tumours [161].

The animal most studied, however, is the golden hamster, since these are the most susceptible. Foci of sarcomatous cells may be found in the kidneys of newborn animals only days after inoculation and they may die after only one or two weeks [338]. With smaller doses death is delayed and tumours may be found in a variety of organs. Older hamsters, too, may develop growths after big doses and after longer delay. Hamsters also develop necrotic, haemorrhagic lesions in their livers [74]; these appear to be the result of proliferative lesions of endothelium of blood-vessels.

The evidence suggests that one virus particle may suffice to initiate a tumour and that growths arise from multiplication of a single infected cell [340]. It is, however, necessary to inject hundreds or thousands of virions in order to produce this result: possibly only a few of the injected particles have the requisite properties: possibly only an occasional one makes contact with a cell at an auspicious moment.

Study of polyoma tumours teaches one very important lesson. It used to be argued that cancer in man could not be caused by viruses, because of the enormous histological varieties of tumours which are known: it was thought that a different virus must cause each of these and that such a vast number of different tumour viruses was inconceivable. It has now been shown quite clearly by cloning experiments that polyoma virions in a single preparation are alike in that any one of them is capable of causing either a carcinoma or a sarcoma in mice, necrosis in a hamster liver or any other of the many tumours which justify us in giving polyoma virus its name. The same general conclusion could be drawn, of course, when the varied potentialities of individual fowl-tumour viruses were revealed.

Simian vacuolating virus: SV 40

Since 1950 monkey kidney cultures have been used in a big way for research into poliomyelitis and in making vaccines against it. In the course of this work there have come to light many indigenous monkey viruses. These have produced characteristic changes in tissue cultures so that it has been possible to recognize and exclude them from vaccines. They have been given serial numbers – simian virus one (SV one) and so on. There was one, however, now called SV 40, which eluded observation until 1960 because it produced no visible effects in the rhesus cultures which were chiefly used: it did, however, do so when tested in kidney cultures from African monkeys of the genus *Cercopithecus* [355]. Later it was found to produce changes also in rhesus testis and human embryonic cultures. These changes consist of vacuolation of cytoplasm of the cells beginning after three to four days.

It soon became obvious that poliomyelitis vaccines, both 'killed' and live but attenuated ones, contained active SV 40 virus. The virus is more resistant to formaldehyde than is poliovirus and had survived the treatment which fully inactivated that. Thus very large numbers of children had inadvertently been given this SV 40 virus. This was disturbing in view of the oncogenic properties of of the virus which were discovered shortly. There is fortunately no evidence at all that people injected with the virus have suffered any ill effects. Antibodies to the virus may, however, be present in their sera, as they are not in the sera of other people: moreover children given vaccines by mouth may pass it out in the faeces. Now that the facts are known it is of course possible to ensure that no contaminated vaccine is used in the future.

SV 40 is a papovavirus and in size, structure and other basic properties it is very similar to polyoma. Virus particles are found in enormous numbers in nuclei of infected green monkey cells: they may be in a random or regular crystalline arrangement. As with polyoma, the virus DNA can infect. When given to monkeys of various genera, the virus can set up an inapparent infection but it has never been known to produce tumours in them. It has now been cultivated in cells of many species, not only those of primates.

In 1961, soon after its discovery, it was found that SV 40 was oncogenic, and, once more, it was the newborn golden hamster which proved to be the susceptible species [98]. Fibrosarcomata developed in the subcutaneous tissues, but only six months or more after injection. In newborns they appeared in nearly 100 per cent of the animals after an average of 200 days, but in a lower percentage and after a longer interval in hamsters one week or one month old. Animals of four months of age did not develop tumours before eighteen months. Even when they appeared later, all the tumours were highly malignant and grew progressively: metastases were frequent in the lungs. Though localization is primarily in subcutaneous tissues, it has been possible in rats to produce tumours in the brains [132]. It is sometimes, not always, possible to recover infectious virus from the tumours in hamsters.

Adenoviruses

Discovery that SV 40 was oncogenic was not very surprising, for it belongs to the papovavirus family, most members of which can cause tumours of one sort or another. It was, however, quite unexpected when Trentin and his colleagues [360] found that one adenovirus serotype, type 12, could produce sarcomata; once again, this was in suckling hamsters. Other types were later found to be oncogenic, too. The tumours are characteristically composed of small closely packed epithelioid cells.

Adenoviruses have been known since 1953 as agents which cause either inapparent infections or relatively mild illnesses, chiefly involving the respiratory tract. They belong to many serological types: at least thirty-one cause human infections, while there are seven simian types and others infecting pigs, mice, dogs, birds and other species. A canine adenovirus is the causative agent of canine hepatitis. All but the avian ones share a common complement-fixing antigen.

Adenoviruses are icosahedral in form, 70–90 nm. in diameter, with 252 surface capsomeres but no outer membrane: their core contains DNA. Most of them will agglutinate red blood cells, especially those of rats. More is known of the structure of their capsids than is the case with other viruses (plates 15, 16). The twenty triangular faces on their surfaces have six capsomeres along each edge. Those at the apices of the capsids have five others adjacent to them and are called pentons: the others have six neighbours touching them and are called hexons. The pentons are complex, having a base and a fibre projecting from it, as shown in the figures. Serological studies reveal that the hexons, pentons and fibres each contain their own antigens [133]. All the adenoviruses grow readily in tissue culture: HeLa cells have been mainly used for the human viruses.

Three serotypes, 12, 18 and 31, are highly oncogenic for baby hamsters, while type 12 produces tumours in rats and mice also. Tumours produced are sarcomata and have appeared in the lungs, subcutaneous tissues and elsewhere. Those caused by type 12 appear between 26 and 216 days after injection. Other adeno-viruses have so far shown no oncogenic properties though they may transform cells *in vitro*, while yet others, including types 3. 7, 14 and 21, are intermediate, producing tumours in smaller numbers of animals and after longer inoculation periods, some-times more than a year. Some simian and avian adenoviruses have also caused tumours in hamsters.

Infectious virus is not recoverable from adenovirus-induced tumours, but, in contrast with what is the case with the polyoma and SV 40 tumours, the specific viral antigen of the fibre has been identified, at least in adenovirus 12 tumours [175]. Another anti-gen (D) may be present also [112].

The oncogenic and non-oncogenic adenoviruses exhibit certain differences in the ratios of the bases which comprise their nucleic acids [143]. Guanine and cytosine together make up only 48–9 per cent of the nucleic-acid bases of the highly oncogenic viruses, while the corresponding figure for the non-oncogenic ones is 56–7 per cent: the weakly oncogenic ones have an intermediate value. It has been suggested that the lower ratio in the case of the oncogenic ones may make it easier for them to become integrated with the nucleic acid of the host cell and that such integration may be concerned in the neoplastic change. Such arguments, be it noted, do not apply to the cases of the polyoma and SV 40 viruses. The differences in base ratios of adenoviruses can be correlated not only with oncogenic powers but with separation into groups on the basis of performance in haemagglutination tests: with the highly oncogenic types 12, 18 and 31 it has been difficult to reveal haemagglutination at all [319].

Discovery of these unsuspected properties in adenoviruses has raised certain problems. Considerable success has been achieved in immunizing against some particularly troublesome human adenoviruses, either with killed vaccines or with live virus given by the mouth in capsules which only dissolve in the gut [58]. In view of the possibility of producing tumours in man, it has been felt unwise at present to continue with such vaccinations, especially as the illnesses which adenoviruses cause are not very serious and, in civilian populations, not very common. Though evidence has been looked for, there is none as yet to indicate that adenoviruses can actually cause human cancers : the possibility has, however, by no means been excluded.

Complementation and hybridization

Some adenoviruses of human origin will not multiply by themselves in cultures of green monkey (*Cercopithecus*) kidneys : the most they can do is to achieve an incomplete cycle with production of some of the T-antigens, to be described in chapter 12. If, however, they are grown in these cells along with SV 40 they *can* replicate and produce complete adenovirus virions : the yield of the SV 40 is not increased. This effect has been referred to as complementation.

It may be mentioned here as another instance of complementation that in many preparations of adenoviruses there are found much smaller particles, only 22–24 nm. across. These are viruses serologically unrelated to adenoviruses, unable to replicate except in the presence of the latter [28, 288]. Though it has been looked for, there is no evidence that their presence is associated with the oncogenicity of the adenoviruses.

In 1964 three groups of workers [174, 290, 306, 315] published evidence of a very remarkable and unexpected finding. Adenovirus type 7 had been passed a number of times in rhesus kidney cultures and these had become, at some point, contaminated by SV 40. They were therefore treated with antiserum against SV 40 and thereby freed from that virus, at least as regards presence of its complete infectious virions. Yet when hamsters developed tumours after injection of this 'purified' virus, they were found to have in their sera antibodies against an SV 40 antigen – its T-antigen, to be dealt with in chapter 12. The cleaned-up virus was then seen to produce this antigen in tissue cultures. Electron micrographs revealed plenty of adenovirus particles but none resembling SV 40. The discovery stimulated a lot of research as a result of which it has now become clear that a sort of hybrid has been produced [291]. Some part of the SV 40 genetic apparatus has become incorporated into that of the adenovirus, the whole being enclosed in an adenovirus capsid. The surface properties of the hybrid are those of the adenovirus but the oncogenic effects are greater than those of the separate 'parents'. Histologically, some of the tumours had characters intermediate between those due to adenoviruses and SV 40, respectively.

It appeared that preparations of the hybrid contained particles of two kinds – ordinary adenovirus 7 and the complex ones. Presence of both of them was necessary for replication in green monkey cultures. On the other hand the adenovirus alone could multiply in human cells but the hybrid could not do so in the absence of ordinary adenovirus. It was next found that to permit the hybrid to grow in human cells it was not necessary to add the homologous type of adenovirus: other types, for instance 2 and 12, would do as well. The progeny which then appeared contained, as before, the complex adenovirus – SV 40 genome, but encased now in the capsid of a different adenovirus type. This was shown by tests using neutralizing antisera against the new helper type (which worked) and against the original type 7 (which didn't).

When the new virus was of a non-oncogenic type it was found that the hybrid particle had nevertheless retained the ability to cause tumours. 'Non-oncogenic virus populations may be converted to those with oncogenic potential: yet phenotypically the virus is unchanged.'

The hybridization revealed in these experiments is particularly unexpected in that the two viruses involved belong to different virus genera, differing from each other in molecular weight, numbers of capsomeres and in other ways. The value of classification of viruses on orthodox lines might even be questioned.

Rapp and Melnick [291] in reviewing the field raise another question: with some adenoviruses it is the presence of the hybrid virus core which confers upon them their oncogenic powers. It is fortunate that tests are available which enable us to recognise a 'bit' of the SV 40 in these viruses. Could it not be that there are other 'bits' of DNA of extraneous origin but at present unrecognizable, which confer similar pathogenic potentialities on other, or even all oncogenic DNA viruses?

11
Cell Transformation by DNA-Viruses

When a virus enters a cell, one of three things may happen. The virus may fail to obtain a foothold and it will then soon disappear. The virus may multiply and the cell be killed. Such cell death seems usually to occur when oncogenic DNA-viruses are being fully replicated, though this is not the case with fowl tumour viruses. Finally there may develop a virus–cell association in which the cells are changed but not killed and the virus is not replicated in the complete infectious state. The cells are said to undergo transformation. Black [40] defines it thus: 'transformation is a heritable change in the properties of a cell, subsequent to virus infection, which is manifested by the loss of the regulatory restraint of its growth potential'. One must distinguish from this state a 'carrier culture' which appears normal yet continues to produce some virus. What happens here is that the majority of cells in the culture are resistant, perhaps being protected by interferon; nevertheless a few are susceptible and these few produce virus and die in the process. They are relatively few, so their fate is not readily apparent. Treatment with antiserum can 'cure' such cultures but has no effect on those which are transformed.

Cells in a transformed culture may or may not have all the properties of a malignant cell. It is best to think of development of malignancy as occurring in a series of steps. Infection by an oncogenic virus can certainly initiate the process. The virus, or what remains of it, may be concerned in causing all the subsequent events or it may merely have initiated a state of unstable equilibrium such that the cell will automatically continue on a 'rake's progress' leading to full malignancy.

Transformation by polyoma

The sequence of events and the properties of transformed cells have been most studied in the case of polyoma. In cultures of mouse embryo cells, this virus multiplies and causes destruction of 80–90 per cent of the cells. With those which survive a carrier culture is set up; and virus multiplication, cell death and cell growth continue together in a steady state [87]. The carrier state can be cured with antiserum and no infectious virus can be recovered from such of the remaining cells as are transformed. There is a variable resistance of the transformed cells to superinfection with fresh polyoma virus.

In hamster cells, in contrast, there is no cell destruction but a low percentage of cells undergoes transformation: no infectious virus is produced and the transformed cells are resistant to superinfection [227, 343]. Many studies have been carried out with a line of cells derived from baby hamster kidney (BHK 21). Like other indefinitely propagable cell lines, this is not free from a tendency to spontaneous neoplastic change; very large numbers of cells will succeed in growing in the hamster's cheek pouch: probably they have taken an early step on the downward path even before infection with polyoma. This virus, however, has a direct action on the cells; it accelerates transformation and other changes in a rapid and dramatic way, making quantitative study relatively easy [343].

Properties of transformed cells: loss of contact inhibition

Transformation is detected by finding colonies of heaped-up cells occurring on a sheet of virus-infected cells in a culture. The cells are no longer regularly orientated, lying parallel to each other, but are randomly arranged, apparently having scrambled all over each other, making a tiny nodule several layers thick. This is due to loss of contact inhibition – a term requiring some explanation. Cells in culture move and can migrate out of an explant. Abercrombie and Heaysman showed in 1954 [1] that when two moving cells came into contact, their ruffled cell-borders were immobilized and cell movement ceased. This they called contact inhibition, and the important observation was made that it was absent in the case of some tumour cells. Another effect, sometimes erroneously included with contact inhibition, has been called by Stoker and Rubin: 'density-dependent inhibition of cell growth in culture' [342]. Presence of a few cells together causes mutual stimulation and helps cell division (feeder effect), but a point is reached when, in the presence of too many cells, multiplication is inhibited. This effect varies independently of contact inhibition of movement, but both kinds of inhibition may be abrogated in the case of transformed cells.

It has been observed [345] that transformed cells show no inhibition of growth when in contact with one another but may still be inhibited by contact with static normal cells. Actively growing normal cells do not inhibit. This finding may have an important bearing on some aspects of tumour growth. Transformed cells can form isolated colonies when grown in a suspending media made from methylcellulose gel or soft agar [229]: normal cells cannot readily do this. Transformed cells, however, are greatly benefited: presumably when separated from normal cells they are no longer subject to growth inhibition. It turns out that use of the sloppy gel technique furnishes a very sensitive method for quantitative study of cell transformation. Colonies of cells developing in the gel can be recognized and counted: they grow more readily than in a cell-sheet.

Thus we may suppose that when, in an animal, less malignant cancer cells are liberated into the blood-stream, they may, if lodging singly in lungs or elsewhere, be so subject to growth inhibition through contact with the normal cells around them that they fail to establish themselves, and so do not grow up into a metastasis. The latent period from inoculation to visible growth of a small number of tumour cells may similarly be explained. First, there is need of a few cells to encourage each other to get started by the feeder effect. Then a focus must be elaborated large enough so that there are cells in its centre no longer in contact with the inhibiting cells around. Stoker suggests that the behaviour of some transformed or malignant cells is to be explained in the light of the idea that these inhibiting mechanisms depend on two factors – the emission of a signal prohibiting cell division or movement and the ability to respond to such a signal. Transformed cells can evidently still receive and respond but have lost their 'transmission sets' [339]. Others may have lost the ability to respond and would thus be able to grow without inhibition. It is possible that a growth inhibitor can be actually transferred from normal to contiguous transformed cells and this may act by inhibiting DNA synthesis [344].

Transplantability

Loss of contact inhibition is a step on the road, but we come nearer to actual neoplastic change in discovering what happens when transformed cells are transplanted into a living host. Cells recently transformed often fail to grow: those passed in culture for some time are more likely to do so. They may at first succeed in establishing themselves only in animals rendered less resistant by X-irradiation, but after passage *in vivo* or *in vitro* they may be able to grow in untreated hosts [82]. This behaviour recalls what happens when one tries to establish a primary tumour in an animal: initially there are difficulties but as further transplantations are carried out, success comes more and more easily. Apparently, there is an increase in malignant potential and autonomy of the cells. As the progression occurs, transplanted cells grow faster, invade more aggressively and produce more metastases. Hamster cells transformed by polyoma, however, though seeming to be highly anaplastic, and growing rapidly, are not highly invasive and do not metastasize freely.

Enders and Diamandopoulos lately reported [103] that a line of cells derived from the heart of a newborn hamster could be transformed by SV 40. Serial passage *in vitro* led to some increased ability to produce lung metastases but to no other dramatic changes. On the other hand a single *in vivo* passage in the tissues of young hamsters caused immediate increase in oncogenic potential: many fewer cells were necessary to cause progressive growth, tumours grew faster and almost all produced visible metastases. The authors inclined to the view that the later changes were due to mutation and selection of cells with new properties rather than to continuing action of the virus.

Morphological changes

Cells transformed by different viruses are different in appearance. Those changed by polyoma are mostly spindle-shaped: SV 40 produces larger, more polygonal cells, while those transformed by adenoviruses look like small epithelial cells with scanty cytoplasm [40]. The adenovirus–SV 40 hybrids may yield tumours with the morphology associated with either 'parent' or something of intermediate appearance may be seen.

Pathologists know very well that there are all sorts of chromosomal abnormalities in cancer cells: and such changes are seen in cells transformed by viruses. They appear, however, to be secondary: loss of contact inhibition, increased transplantability and other changes appear before chromosomal abnormalities. It is true that these are seen more and more as the cells show signs of increasing malignancy, but it would be rash to speculate as to what is cause and what is effect.

Other effects of transformation

The appearance of new antigen in transformed cells is a matter of great interest, but this will be dealt with in the next chapter.

DNA-viruses have the power of stimulating DNA synthesis in infected cells and this seems to be accomplished by catalysing the formation of at least six enzymes concerned in the production of DNA [40]. The question arises of whether the manufacture of naturally occurring host enzymes is stimulated or whether the virus genome is able to code for the production of its own enzymes. The results are conflicting, but there is evidence that at least one enzyme which appears has properties differing from those of the normal host cell [198]. The DNA which is formed is apparently of host origin: little or no viral DNA is made when the association between virus and cell does not involve production of new virus.

Disappearance and rescue of virus

It has already been pointed out that in most instances no infectious virus can be released by ordinary techniques from cells transformed by DNA-viruses. In the case of the mouse-cell–polyoma system this is evident, once the transformed cells have been freed from mixture with cells in the carrier-culture state which may be present also. Nor can the antigen of the virions be detected except in the instance of the fibre virion in cultures transformed by adenovirus 12 [175]. It will, however, be shown that other antigens, the T and transplantation antigens, are regularly present, so that some part of the virus or a virus-footprint must remain.

No way of rescuing complete polyoma or adenovirus has been described, though experiments with SV 40 suggest that this may yet be achieved. When apparently virus-free cells transformed by SV 40 are cultivated along with normal green monkey cells, either primary cultures or lines derived from them, infectious virus can once more be extracted [42, 130]. This result recalls those reported in chapter 6, when Rous virus could be rescued from apparently virus-free Rous tumours in mammals by cultivation along with normal chicken cells. As in that instance, rescue is greatly helped with the SV 40 cells if inactivated Sendai virus is present. This seems to operate, first, by opening up intercellular bridges between adjacent cells and then by causing their complete fusion. We do not know just how the green monkey cell is able to rescue the virus. The cell-fusion technique has not been successful in rescuing virus from all lines of cells transformed by SV 40. On the other hand, in a few instances it has been possible to obtain a little free virus by means other than cell fusion – by treatment with mitomycin, proflavine or hydrogen peroxide [42]. The findings suggest an analogy with the induction of bacteriophage by treatment of lysogenic bacteria with ultra-violet radiation or in other ways : most workers, however, feel that the analogy is not so very close [206].

Mechanism of transformation

Clearly, the virus DNA is the active agent in causing cell transformation and one naturally enquires whether there is anything remarkable about it which makes this feat possible. In papovaviruses, the DNA may be circular or linear and it appears that only circular DNA is particularly effective. It appears that only a part of the virus genome is necessary to effect transformation : X-irradiation in a dose which destroys infectivity does not remove its ability to transform. There is evidence suggesting that the virus DNA may actually be inserted into chromosomes of host-cells, and this is a useful working hypothesis. Much interest accordingly attaches to reports that transformation may be reversible, for it would hardly be expected that pieces of virus DNA could keep jumping in and out of host chromosomes. It has been shown [228] that in hamster cultures transformed by the SR strain of Rous virus, 'revertants' may appear. This is not very surprising, since the Rous virus grows in the cytoplasm and the question of integration into host genomes does not arise. Possibly the virus genome is not replicated sufficiently fast and gets lost by being diluted out. The revertant colonies are not quite normal, since their cells are resistant to renewed transformation by the virus.

One wonders how to interpret Stoker's [341] experiments on 'abortive transformation' by polyoma. He found that many cells of the hamster line BHK 21 when grown in a special (methocel) suspending medium could undergo a number of divisions after infection with polyoma, considerably more than in the absence of virus. They no longer needed, as normal cells do, anchorage to a solid base in order to be able to multiply progressively: thus they had acquired at least one property of transformed cells and there are suggestions that they may have gained others, too. Only a few of the micro-colonies, however, went on to become fully transformed. Most reverted and ceased to continue to grow in suspension. It seems very unlikely that this first stage in progression to transformation and perhaps malignancy can have been mediated by integration of the virus's genome into that of the host cells. Reversion of cells fully transformed by polyoma has also been accomplished [231].

SV 40 and human cells

SV 40 is one of the few viruses which has as yet been shown to be able to transform human cells [208]. Many of the experiments have been carried out with WI-38, one of the lines of human cells developed at the Wistar Institute in Philadelphia. Many cell-lines under study in laboratories come from cancers or have developed malignant characters: they have chromosomal abnormalities and can be carried indefinitely in culture. These Wistar lines on the other hand have normal chromosomes and normally die out after some forty to fifty cell divisions. They are sufficiently free from suspicions of malignancy to have been proposed for use in making virus-vaccines for man. It is interesting that when they cease to grow well at the end of their career, it is far easier to transform them with SV 40 than at an earlier stage. In contrast to what is found with cells from most other species [82], human cells infected with SV 40 continue for long periods to yield infectious virus. Yet this does not go on indefinitely. For a time only a few cells shed virus, but these few shed quite a lot. Later all are found to be shedders, yet each yields only comparatively few virus particles, and still later virus production may cease altogether [321]. The cultures have been observed to go through a period of crisis when growth seems to be grinding to a halt: it may be like the dying-out which occurs in uninfected cultures. In the infected cultures a few cells seem to survive and these eventually start growing again as fully transformed cells, free from infectious virus.

One would naturally like to know whether human cells transformed by SV 40 are truly malignant. One cannot, of course, inject them into normal persons, and in any case they might not grow, as even with rodents it is desirable to use closely inbred animals for such tests. However, such cultures have been injected into patients who already have cancer and are unlikely to survive for very long. In them the SV 40-treated cultures have produced nodules which have the histological appearances of sarcomata: they have all regressed spontaneously [134]. One must not draw conclusions too readily from such experiments: the very fact that the patients already had cancers may mean that their resistance was unlike that of normal people.

12
New Tumour Antigens

There exists an extensive, confusing and often contradictory literature on immunological aspects of cancer. Fortunately, work on the
antigens associated with virus tumours has been able to throw
some light on the darkness. Newly discovered tumour antigens are
of at least two kinds. There are the T-antigens, formerly called
neo-antigens, mainly present in cell nuclei and recognized by the
use of the complement-fixation test or with the help of antibody
rendered fluorescent by being tagged with a fluorescent dye. In
contrast, are transplantation antigens. These are concerned with
the rejection of transplants by immune hosts and may also be detected in tests for cytotoxicity: such tests may usefully be carried
out by seeing whether serum or cells from an immune animal will
inhibit the formation of colonies of tumour cells in cultures. The
transplantation antigens are present on the surface of transformed
or malignant cells.

T-antigens

Huebner and his colleagues showed [173] that hamsters bearing
primary or transplanted tumours caused by an adenovirus had
complement-fixing antibodies in their sera: these reacted with
extracts of the tumours but not with the adenovirus virions. They
did, however, show considerable specificity: the sera from hamsters with tumours caused by adenovirus type 12 cross-reacted
only with antigens of the other two highly oncogenic viruses, types
18 and 31. The antigens of these three viruses thus fell into one
antigenic group while those of the moderately oncogenic ones (3,
7, 14, 21) [178] shared another, distinct, antigen. These antigens, called T- (tumour-) antigens, had thus novel properties: they
were virus-specific yet not detectable in the mature virus particle.

It was soon shown that similar T-antigens were present in tumours caused by SV 40 and polyoma viruses: these, again, had their own specificity. In tumours caused by SV 40–adenovirus hybrids, the T-antigens of both viruses were frequently present [291]. This suggests that the T-antigens were coded for by the virus's own nucleic acid, not by that of the cell, for the same ones were present in tumour cells of mice, hamsters or other species so long as they were caused by the same virus.

The antigens have been found not only in tumours: they are regularly present also in cells transformed by viruses in culture and their continued presence, as indicated earlier, is one of the characters by which transformation is recognized. They are more heat-labile than are virus antigens and are less readily sedimented in the centrifuge. Those of polyoma and SV 40 can be located in the nuclei of cells by staining with fluorescent antibody, while those of adenovirus tumours are apparently present both in nucleus and cytoplasm and they may be arranged as bundles of fibrous protein.

Though transformation does not seem to occur unless T-antigens are formed, presence of this antigen is not the only thing necessary to lead to that result. Many cells contain the antigen, yet lose it after a few cell divisions and fail to be transformed [41]. In fact it now appears that during any infection of cells by oncogenic viruses, T-antigen regularly appears, though perhaps only transiently [314]. It can be detected after six to ten hours, before any infectious virus appears. The suggestion has been made that the T-antigen is an enzyme having a function early in the course of synthesis of new virions, normally disappearing at a later stage. It has not, however, been identified as yet as corresponding to any previously known enzyme. It may well be that in cells which are abortively infected, the later stages of virus synthesis cannot be accomplished and that persistent production of T-antigen is a corollary. There are known to be 'early proteins' which appear early in the course of infection of cells by viruses which are not oncogenic [172]: they are not detectable at later stages. In the non-oncogenic virus infections they are never known to persist.

Antibodies against T-antigen increase in titre as tumours grow. If the tumours are excised, they decrease or disappear, but may reappear if the tumours recur [173]. Their theoretical interest is considerable, especially since they afford some of the best evidence that a part of the virus's genome must persist though infectivity is lost. There is, however, no evidence that their presence is related to resistance to tumour growth. The other kind of antigen, transplantation antigen, is here of greater interest.

Transplantation antigens

These were discovered before the T-antigens. Sjögren and his colleagues [330] and Habel [155] independently showed that adult mice immunized with polyoma virus would reject transplants of polyoma-caused tumours, other than very large ones, even though the experiments were carried out in genetically homogeneous mice. It has also proved possible to immunize mice by injection of 'virus-free' tumours, using material from genetically different mice so that the immunizing tumour cells would not themselves grow. There is abundant evidence that the immunity is unrelated to the presence of antiviral antibodies. Further, the transplantation immunity varies independently of antibody to T-antigen. There are various differences between 'transplantation antigen' and the T-antigen system, besides similarities. The transplantation antigens are evidently on the surface of cells, not in the nucleus. They are virus-specific but rather less so than in the case of T-antigens: thus there is some crossing between adenoviruses of the high and low oncogenic groups: and there is even a report of slight crossing between the antigens of SV 40 and a human papilloma virus [236]. As with T-antigens, all tumours caused by one strain of virus have the same transplantation antigen, but, in contrast to T-antigen, this is true only where a single species is concerned: mouse polyoma virus is relatively inefficient in protecting hamsters against injection of polyoma-transformed hamster cells. This species difference is, however, not seen in cytotoxic tests involving the inhibition of colony formation in culture.

Sjögren has suggested that presence of a strange antigen on the cell surface, abolition of contact inhibition and other changes seen in transformed or malignant cells may all be manifestations of a single change in surface structure.

An important aspect of transplantation-resistance is that cellular mechanisms are more effective than humoral ones. Resistance to transplantation of polyoma tumours is readily transferred by means of lymphocytes of immune animals, not with serum [8]. Thymectomy, which is particularly damaging to cell-mediated immunity, greatly reduces the resistance of mice to polyoma, so that they will develop tumours at an age when they would otherwise be resistant [216]. Mention was made earlier of the spontaneous appearance of tumours in a polyoma-contaminated environment among thymectomized mice. There are good reasons to believe that polyoma virus produces tumours as a rule only in very small mice, just because their cellular immunity has not had time to develop : probably it does so more slowly than the humoral mechanism. This, rather than immunological tolerance is likely to be the factor concerned [8]. The same argument applies to the susceptibility of very young animals to other oncogenic viruses. Special factors apply in the case of mouse leukaemia viruses which grow in thymic tissue and may fail to cause leukaemia in thymectomized animals. The role of cellular immunity will be further discussed in chapter 19 with special reference to the picture in man.

The transplantation antigen, like the T-antigen, appears in cells transformed in culture. It may, however, disappear from such cells when they have been carried in culture for a long time. It was shown in the case of an SV 40-caused hamster tumour that the transplantation antigen was lost and that this loss coincided with the ability of the tumour to metastasize : no antigen could be detected in the metastatic nodules [77]. One can readily see that there might be a connection between successful implantation of a metastasis and failure to reject a tumour transplant.

A surprising finding has been that repeated inoculation of an oncogenic virus, instead of favouring the development of tumours may be actually inhibitory [283]. Thus, in one experiment, cancer appeared in 50 per cent of newborn hamsters inoculated with SV 40 virus. If, however, *after* their first virus inoculation, more SV 40 was repeatedly injected, the incidence was reduced to less than 5 per cent. Similar experiments are on record with polyoma and adenovirus type 12.

In another type of experiment, adult hamsters with transplanted SV 40 tumours had their tumours excised, after which they were repeatedly injected with SV 40 virus [85]. This treatment greatly reduced the incidence of recurrences. In all these experiments the effects were specific: unrelated viruses achieved nothing: nor did homologous killed virus. It appears that a tumour antigen, potentially useful as an immunizing agent, may be so closely associated with a growing tumour that it is unable to induce any immunity, yet virus injected during the latent period before a tumour becomes visible may, if in large enough quantity, evoke an antigenic response. Possibly it achieves this by causing some transformation or abortive transformation of many cells, leading to production of tumour antigens which can immunize. It is not necessary to inject infectious virus: the same result is attained by injecting irradiated tumours or tumours which will not grow because coming from a genetically different host [273]. A course of injections of irradiated SV 40 tumours could thus prevent the development of SV 40 tumours in baby hamsters or would inhibit takes of transplants of SV 40 tumours in adult hamsters. Disrupted tumour tissue was useless. In contrast, tumours caused by adenovirus 7 could be broken up by alternate freezing and thawing or in other ways and would still immunize. This sort of experiment suggests a possible method of treating cancers in man and particularly in preventing metastases or recurrences after operation: a 'vaccine' could be made from removed tumour tissue. It must be confessed that though treatment in this sort of way has been attempted over many years, success in human cancers has been negligible. This may be because, as is now known, specific antigens in most naturally occurring tumours are either absent or unique for each particular growth. Possibly, however, technical modifications, based on the experiments with virus tumours, may lead to better results in the future.

13

Warts in Rabbits and Other Species

A number of papovaviruses cause warts or papillomas in their mammalian hosts. With a few exceptions, to be mentioned below, they are specific for their natural hosts, or at most infect a few closely related species. In their behaviour they are intermediate between the poxviruses and the fowl-tumour viruses. Unlike the poxes, the cell proliferations they produce persist for months or even for the lifetime of the host, but progression to malignancy is far from being the general rule: they are normally innocent growths. So much is known now about the rabbit papilloma virus that it will be discussed in detail, with briefer mention of the other wart viruses.

Papillomatosis of rabbits

R. E. Shope described in 1933 an 'infectious papillomatosis of rabbits' [324]. He had been told that in north-western Iowa hunters frequently shot cottontail rabbits (*Sylvilagus floridanus*) bearing horn-like protuberances on the skin. These he obtained and warty rabbits were later procured from elsewhere in the USA. The warts did not seem to trouble the animals: one, however, was covered with them and material obtained post-mortem 'was sufficient to fill a 200-c.c. flask'. The warts frequently had a pale fleshy centre but projecting parts were hard, keratinized, blackish and vertically striated. One horn six inches long has been recorded. Of naturally occurring growths in cottontails 21 per cent regressed within six months and 36 per cent within the following eighteen months. When there are multiple warts, regression occurs in all of them together. Rabbits in which regression has occurred are not necessarily wholly resistant to reinfection.

Shope had no difficulty in transmitting warts with glycerolated material both to cottontails and to domestic rabbits, when this was rubbed into lightly scarified skin (plate 17). The inoculation period was very variable: eight days was an average time. The warts produced resembled the naturally occurring ones except that regression was less frequent. It was soon shown that filtrates were active and that sera of infected rabbits had neutralizing and complement-fixing antibodies active against the virus. Filtrates were inactive when inoculated otherwise than by skin scarification: the virus was unusually heat-stable, surviving heating for thirty minutes at 67° C. Subsequent work has added greatly to knowledge of the virus's properties. It is now known to be a DNA-containing virus belonging to the papovaviruses. Like the other wart viruses, it is rather larger than are polyoma and SV 40, having a diameter of 42–54 nm. As is the case with others of this family, there is dispute as to the number of capsomeres: figures of forty-two, sixty, seventy-two and ninety-two have been put forward. Perhaps the most convincing is the claim of Finch and Klug [115] that the virus is an icosahedron of left-handed skew form with seventy-two capsomeres. Abnormal elongated forms have been described. Growth apparently begins in the nucleolus but soon the whole nucleus may be involved, and within it virus particles may be found in more or less orderly array.

The double-stranded DNA of the virus is circular and perhaps 2·3 to 2·8 μ long. Phenol extraction of virus preparations has yielded DNA which is infectious. It might be expected that active virus would be most readily obtained from the lower actively proliferating layers of the stratified epithelium: on the contrary, fluorescent antibody reveals that antigen is mainly present in the more superficial keratinizing layers of the wart [262].

Attempts have been made to grow the virus in tissue or organ cultures of rabbit skin. Most workers have failed to demonstrate serial passage of the virus in the ordinary way but the virus-treated cells have given rise to tumours when introduced into the cheek-pouches of hamsters [210].

Osato and Ito [272] tried to grow the virus in rabbit cells at

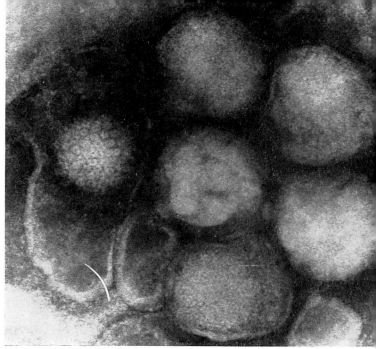

1 Electron micrograph of herpes virus virions. The left-hand
one clearly shows, within the membrane, the nucleocapsid
with its regularly arranged capsomeres. ×300,000.

2 Herpes-type intranuclear inclusion bodies in culture of
calf thyroid cells infected with bovine malignant catarrh
virus. ×1700.

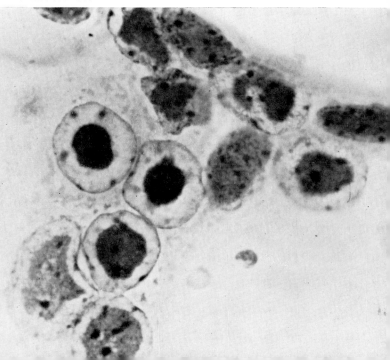

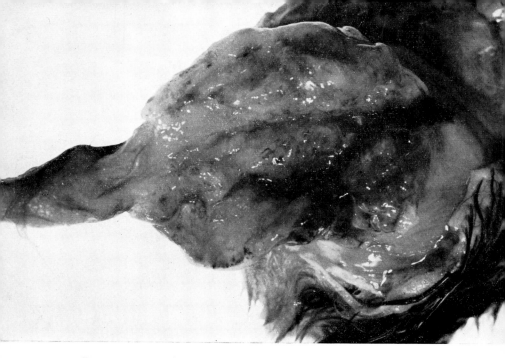

3 Rous sarcoma induced by virus in the leg muscle of a chicken. ×4.

4 Section of Rous sarcoma in a chicken, showing spindle cells, myxomatous stroma and a lymphoid nodule. ×400.

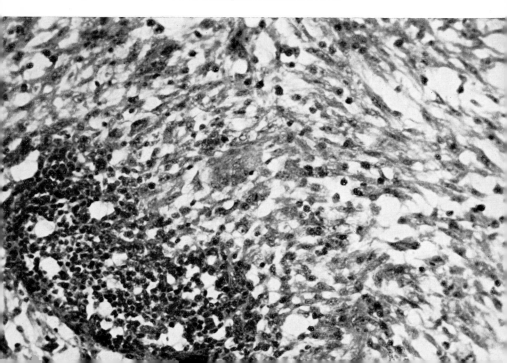

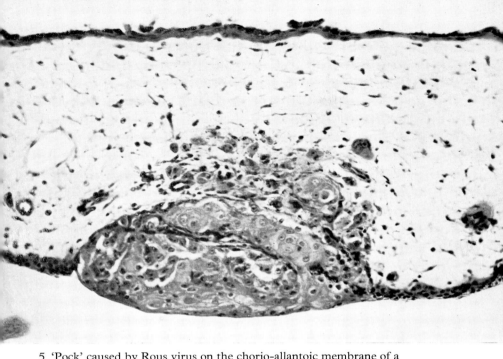

5 'Pock' caused by Rous virus on the chorio-allantoic membrane of a developing egg. Ectodermal proliferation and some involvement of mesoderm. ×335.

6 Foci of transformed cells produced nine days after infection of chicken embryo fibroblasts with Rous sarcoma virus. Phase-contrast. ×120.

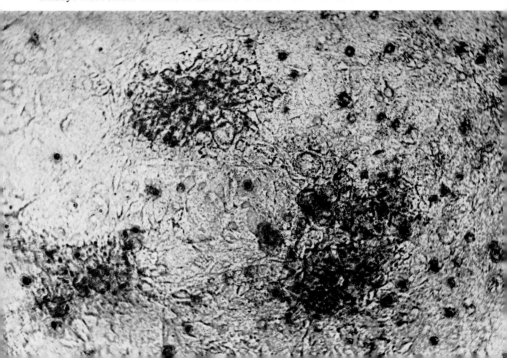

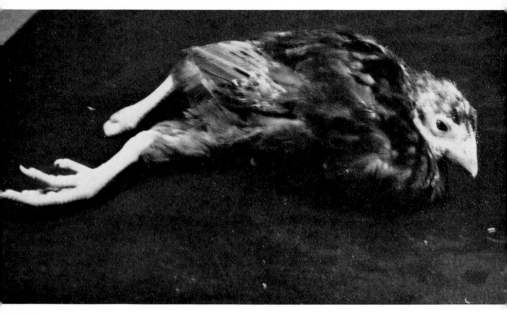

7 Chicken paralysed as a result of infection with Marek's disease.

8 Section through nerve of a chick paralysed by Marek's disease, showing infiltration of the nerve with masses of small round cells.

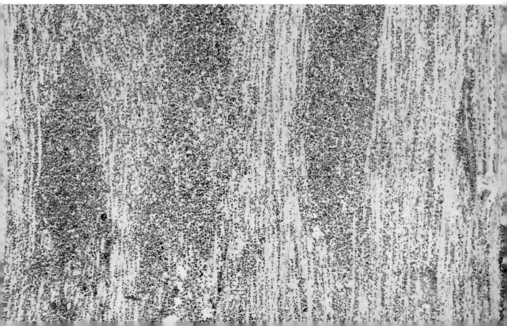

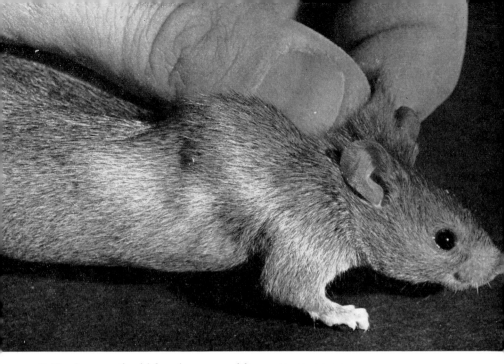

9 Twelve-month-old female mouse with spontaneous mammary tumour. ×2.

10 Section through a spontaneous mammary tumour in a mouse. ×255.

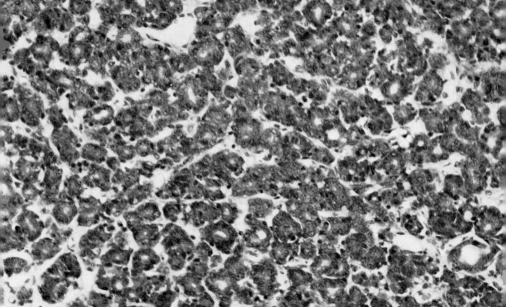

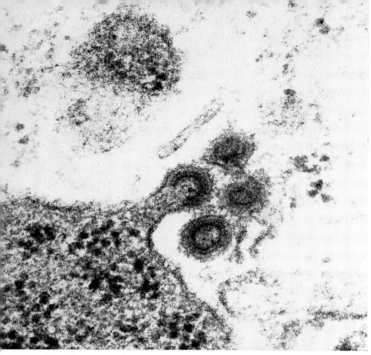

11 Electron-microscopic picture of a section through a mouse lymphoma induced by Moloney virus, showing C-type particles, one of them budding off from the surface of a tumour cell. ×200,000.

12 Section through the cheek-pouch of a hamster inoculated twenty days previously with a human breast cancer. ×100.

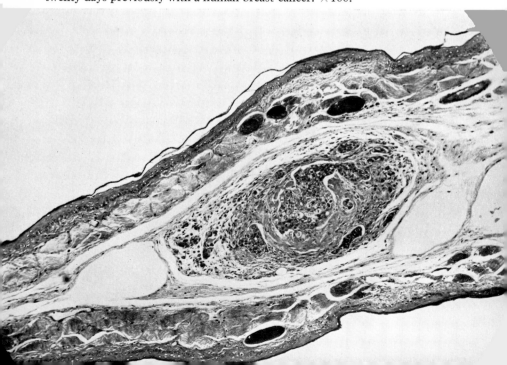

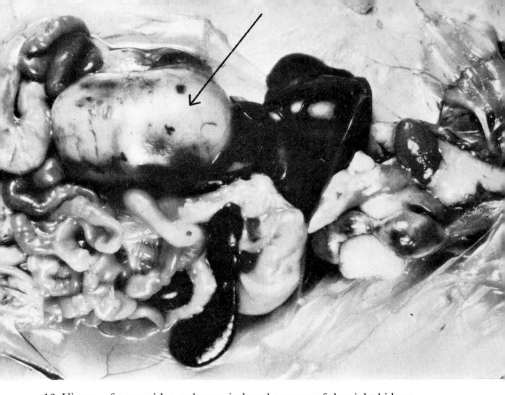

13 Viscera of a rat with a polyoma-induced tumour of the right kidney and chest wall (indicated by arrow).

14 Purified and fractionated polyoma virus particles. ×280,000.

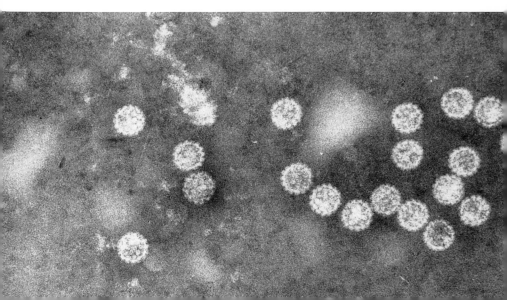

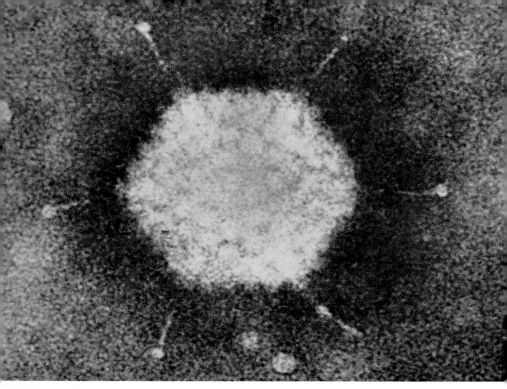

15 Electron micrograph of an adenovirus, showing fibres at the apices of the icosahedron. ×800,000.

16 Diagram of an adenovirus virion showing the constituent elements.

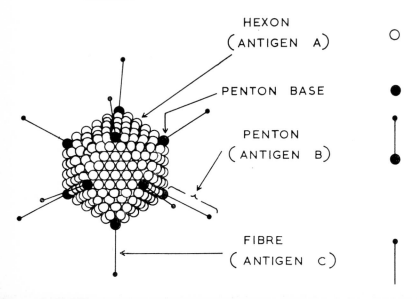

HEXON
(ANTIGEN A)

PENTON BASE

PENTON
(ANTIGEN B)

FIBRE
(ANTIGEN C)

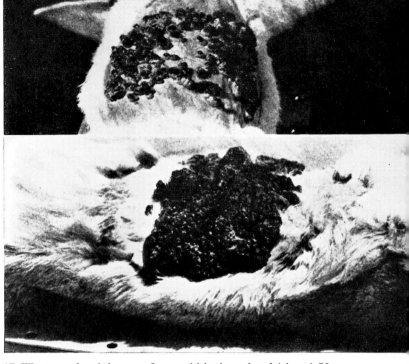

17 Warts on the abdomen of two rabbits inoculated (above) 52 days and (below) 118 days previously with papilloma virus.

18 Warts on the flank of a rabbit which have undergone malignant change and have formed, below, an indurated mass.

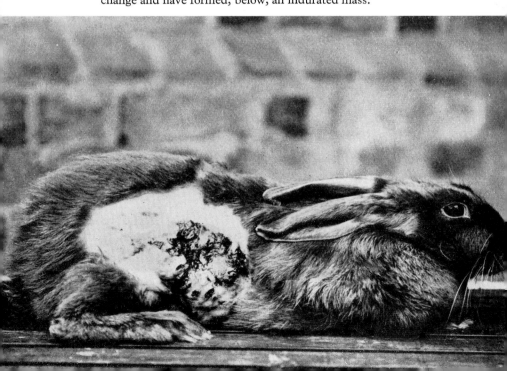

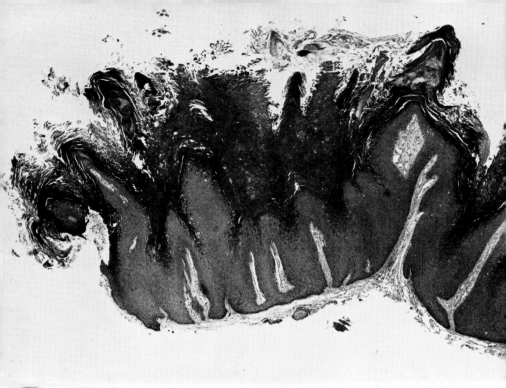

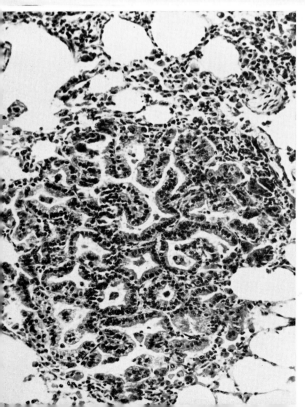

19 Section through a human wart, showing proliferation of epithelium and (above) over-production of horny material (keratin). ×45.

20 Jaagsiekte (pulmonary adenomatosis) of sheep. Section of a small focal lesion in the lung, showing alveoli lined mainly with columnar epithelium. ×210.

21 Spontaneous growth on the face of a rhesus monkey caused by Yaba virus.

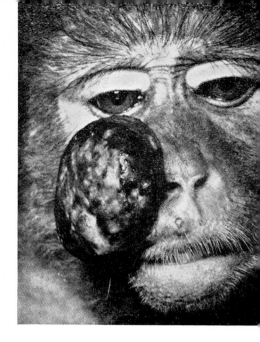

22 Electron micrograph of virions of molluscum contagiosum. × 18,000.

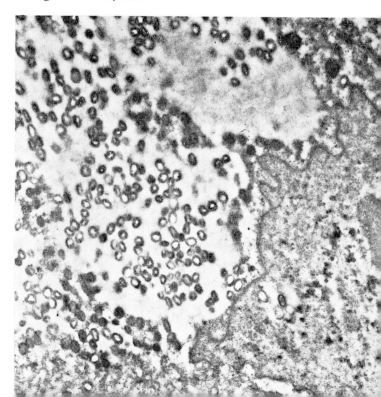

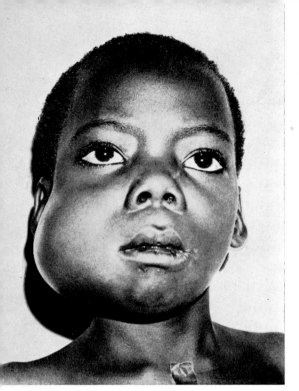

23 African boy with a mandibular (Burkitt) tumour.

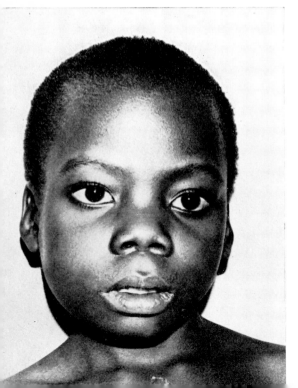

24 The same boy fourteen days later, following an injection of cyclophosphamide.

37° C. and examined their cultures with fluorescent anti-body. Virus was detected in the nucleus but the fluorescent cells diminished in numbers and soon were seen no more. They then reflected that the surface of the rabbit's skin was probably much cooler than 37° C., so they transferred these non-staining cultures to 30° C., and found that staining in the cells quickly reappeared: this time, however, it was the cytoplasm which stained. Similar findings were reported by Shiratori [322]. It is possible that it was the rabbit vacuolating virus (see p. 90) which was activated in these experiments.

One very important observation was made by Shope. Although the virus infected domestic rabbits as readily as it did cottontails, things were very different when it came to recovering virus for serial passage. It was commonly impossible to recover infectious virus from these warts and serial passage in domestic rabbits was rarely achieved. Shope did, in one series, achieve fourteen such passes in series but this result was exceptional. The occasional successes are less significant than the usual failure. It was suggested that in domestic rabbit warts enough antibody seeped in to neutralize the virus's activity, but this explanation carried no conviction. Shope then showed that extracts of non-infectious warts injected into rabbits intraperitoneally would immunize and provoke the appearance of specific antibodies. He argued that virus might be present in a 'masked' form. This idea of masking of virus provoked considerable controversy. Beard [34] succeeded in purifying the virus and argued that the difference between cottontail warts and tame rabbit warts was a purely quantitative one, the former containing at least 200 times as much virus as the latter: he also showed that antibodies could be induced with much less virus than was required to cause warts. His arguments were cogent, but it nevertheless appears that Shope was in the main right after all. As has been shown for other tumours caused by papovaviruses, there are antigens and antibodies other than those concerned with the virion. Kidd [190], studying the regression of warts, observed that this occurred as a result of an immunity process independent of virus-neutralizing antibody and thought it likely that this was due to immunity directed against tumour cells rather than virus. There is now suggestive evidence that the warts

D

may contain a T-antigen similar to that described for polyoma and other virus tumours [373]. Thus, Beard may well have explained correctly why wart suspensions can evoke antibodies in the apparent absence of infectious virus: but Shope was correct in his surmise that virus may exist in warts in an incomplete form. The terms masked or occult can be used: Shope later suggested [325] that virus might be there as infectious DNA, and if the genome persists, DNA must be present, though things may be more complex than was first thought.

Apart from the very important question of masking, the rabbit papilloma is of great interest because of the questions of the relation of warts to malignant tumours and the progression of many warts to malignancy. Before discussing this it is well to review what is known of the wart viruses of other mammals.

Warts in man

Warts of many kinds are described in man, and many of them are due to an infectious virus [308] (plate 19). There are juvenile or plane warts, digitate, filiform, plantar, genital and laryngeal warts. It has been suggested that they are fundamentally of two different kinds, which respectively are and are not associated with presence of intranuclear inclusions [223]. Solid evidence, however, only concerns those due to a papovavirus, and this does form inclusions in infected cells. The basophilic ones consist largely of virus particles, often arranged in a very regular manner, but eosinophilic inclusions may be due to abnormal keratinization. The human papilloma virus is structurally like that of the rabbit virus: according to Klug and Finch [205] it is a skew icosahedron but the skew, in contrast to the rabbit virus, is right-handed. As with the rabbit virus, the infectious virions are mainly present in the superficial keratinized layers of the warts. Antibodies against the virus have been demonstrated by double diffusion in agar and other techniques; they are not present in all people with warts. When infection is deliberately transmitted from man to man, the incubation period is said to vary between six weeks and twenty months: a period of two to six months is commonest. The 'condyloma acuminatum' of the genital region is probably due to the same virus: this form of wart may occasionally become malignant.

Infectious warts in man may persist for months but tend ultimately to regress. They are rather readily cured by cautery or other destructive measures. Their sudden spontaneous disappearance is believed to be due to development of immunity and it is likely that this is similar to that occurring against rabbit warts. Its unpredictable occurrence has increased the reputation of various folk-lore remedies, but it is not easy to discredit the claims for cure by means of hypnosis.

Papillomatosis of cattle and other ungulates

In contrast to the warts of rabbit and man, those of cattle have a large element of connective tissue proliferation in them [136]. They are not strictly species-specific and have caused connective tissue tumours on transmission to horses [268], newborn hamsters and one strain of mice [45]. The virus has been cultivated in fertile hens' eggs [269]. It has also proved capable of transforming embryonic hamster cells *in vitro*. The transformed cells gave rise to serially propagable tumours in the hamsters [129]. It resembles that of other wart viruses morphologically. The warts in cattle may be present in enormous numbers, especially on the head or neck, persisting for months before they regress: they may apparently be responsible also for bladder-growths in cattle.

The fibroma virus of deer causes multiple tumours in the North American white-tailed deer. They are very similar to the growths in cattle but could not be transmitted to a calf [326].

Equine papillomatosis affects chiefly the nose and lips, and is due to a similar virus, infecting only horses [67]. It is not known whether the connective tissue tumours or 'sarcoids' found in horses are due to the same virus; they may even be caused by the bovine virus.

Little is known of the papillomatosis of sheep and goats. It is said that the warts may become malignant.

Papillomatosis of other species

An oral papillomatosis may be troublesome in young dogs and is due to a papovavirus: dermal warts in dogs may be due to a different virus. The oral virus has not been transmitted to other species.

Warts in South American *Cebus* monkeys have been transmitted to old and new-world monkeys of several species.

There is a virus causing oral papillomatosis of domestic rabbits [275]. This is quite distinct from Shope's cottontail virus and affects only mucous membranes; it can be transmitted experimentally to *Sylvilagus* and *Lepus* species. Warts in hamsters may be due to yet another virus. Finally, mention should be made of a rabbit kidney vacuolating virus, present as a latent infection in cottontail rabbits; it is due to a papovavirus [163], is not known to cause tumours of any sort, but is mentioned as it has led to confusion in some experiments with the rabbit papillomatosis virus.

Shope's rabbit papilloma is of much interest because of the apparent disappearance of the virus from the warts in domestic rabbits. Even more important are the findings concerning the malignant changes which supervene spontaneously both in cottontails and tame rabbits. Before these are described, it is well to look at some work published by Rous and Beard in 1934 [297]: this reveals that the straightforward warts themselves have unexpected malignant potential [cf also 305]. Papillomatosis material was taken from rabbits with precautions to avoid bacterial contamination, finely minced and injected into the same rabbits' muscles or, after laparotomy, into various viscera. The wart tissue not only survived but grew progressively, causing at times enormous growths from which the animals commonly died. Growth was faster in cottontails, one dying after thirty-nine, another after eighty-one days: the tumours went forward more slowly in the tame rabbits. While all this was happening, the remaining superficial warts remained stationary or even regressed.

Some of the visceral tumours were encapsulated, others not: blunt papillomatous processes could be seen penetrating into surrounding tissues: there might or might not be a surrounding cellular reaction. At times there was widespread interstitial cellulitis in injected muscles and then: 'the papilloma ... showed an active malignancy, sending out long, thin, disorderly tongues of proliferating epithelial cells which thrust between and around the individual muscle fibres'. Intravenous injection of small cell fragments led to the growth of embolic papillomata in the lungs and

these showed invasive properties: there was, however, no conclusive evidence of metastasis from the growths which developed
in muscles or viscera.

Rous and Beard failed to pass these growths in series. Later,
however, Rogers [292], working in Rous' laboratory, was successful in achieving this, provided that he used suckling rabbits. In
some of these the growths did well, forming large masses, even at
times after the hosts had matured. They even 'penetrated the re-
active tissue encapsulating them and replaced the adjacent muscle'
but they 'never metastasized nor did they undergo carcinomatous
change'. Even when the inoculated baby rabbits had grown up,
their growths could not be transplanted into adults.

The question naturally arose of why the skin warts did not
normally behave as malignant growths. Beard and Rous [35] were
able to modify their behaviour. Injection under them of the dyes
Scharlach R or Sudan III caused a temporary malignancy, so that
the affected epithelium began to burrow downwards. When, however, the Scharlach R had had time to disappear, the effect was no
longer seen and the growths became quiescent. Similar down-
growing invasive growth was induced by covering newly appearing
warts with collodion so that they could not grow outwards but had
perforce to grow inwards. Rous and Beard [297] conclude that
the papilloma 'often looks and acts like a malignant neoplasm . . .
The morphology and behaviour of the generality of tumours can
no longer be held to exclude the possibility that these are produced
by extraneous living entities.'

Before all this work was concluded Shope had reported to Rous
that a domestic rabbit inoculated with the virus 393 days earlier
had developed 'an epidermoid carcinoma of unequivocal malignancy'. It soon appeared that this was no unusual occurrence:
many persisting papillomata went on to become malignant (plate
18), and this occurred in cottontails, too, though far less frequently
than in domestic rabbits. Peyton Rous and his colleagues carried
out a number of important studies of the carcinomas [298]. It
appeared that the cancerous change was more apt to appear after a
large inoculation of papilloma virus leading to rapid and extensive
growth and when such a growth had persisted for a considerable
time. The original tumour always remained constant in its form

until malignancy occurred. But then changes came one after another in different parts of the growth, so that the histological
appearances were very diverse from one area to another [356].
The original benign growth might persist locally or even regress,
but in general the change was always to something more and more
anaplastic. It seemed that quite a small change in the virus was
necessary to tip the scale from innocence to malignancy but that
once a change had begun, the growths entered on a state of unstable equilibrium, so that fresh changes readily occurred. One
could perhaps interpret these as being due to successive somatic
mutations in the cells, or alternatively as mutations in the virus.
If, however, the findings are to be explained on the same lines as
for the tumours caused by polyoma and SV 40 viruses, it seems
that both things may be partly true.

Since infectious virus is obtained with difficulty from tame
rabbit warts, it is not surprising that the cancers, too, fail to yield
any. Yet virus has at times been obtained even from anaplastic
cancers in tame rabbits and much more frequently from those in
cottontails. When this has happened, the virus obtained behaves
just like ordinary papilloma virus: there is no evidence of the
existence of an infectious, immediately carcinogenic, virus.

Most of the rabbit cancers have been transplanted with difficulty to other rabbits: this is doubtless largely because inbred
strains of rabbits have not been available. It has fortunately proved
relatively easy, however, to pass the tumour cells in series through
newborn rabbits, and several lines of transplantable tumours have
thus been obtained. When unaltered papilloma virus has been
recovered from these, it does not follow that this has been responsible for urging on the malignant cells: it may well be that this
virus is merely a passenger, as many other viruses are known to
be passengers in many other tumours. There may well exist, however, independently of such passenger virus, other papilloma
genomes closely associated with cells and these may be playing a
significant role in the malignancy.

Such an explanation is rendered probable by the results of
immunological studies. In one line of transplanted cancer cells, the
VX2 carcinoma, virus was apparently present in small quantity,
or in masked form, for the tumour-bearing rabbits were immune to

infection with papilloma virus and had neutralizing and complement-fixing antibodies in their blood. This state of affairs persisted while transplantations were carried out throughout eight years. Then, at the forty-sixth transplant generation and later, it was found that the rabbits were fully susceptible to virus and had no antibodies in their sera [300]. The tumours behaved in the same manner after the virus had 'disappeared'. Other transplant lines of the tumour have, however, continued to show presence of the virus, as did the VX2 for so many years. It is difficult to avoid the conclusion that presence of some papilloma virus as a passenger is an irrelevancy as far as the behaviour of the cancer is concerned.

Pulmonary adenomatosis in sheep

This is a condition very different from papillomatosis but it is convenient to mention it here. The disease has been known especially from Iceland and South Africa; in the latter country it is known as jaagsiekte, a name meaning driving sickness, since the animals exhibit shortness of breath when driven. The nodules of adenoma, or growths of epithelial cells, grow progressively and come to occupy a large part of the lungs (plate 20). The causative agent has been cultivated in sheep macrophages [226] and intranuclear inclusion bodies have been found, resembling those of herpes [332]. It remains to be established whether the causative agent is, in fact, a herpes virus. In Peru and Israel [261] the disease behaves like a malignant tumour and metastases have been found in lymph-nodes and elsewhere: in other countries this has not been observed.

14
Poxviruses

All the viruses of the pox group give rise to cell proliferation at an early stage of the infection. The overgrowth of tissue thus produced is, however, self-limited. After a time there is regression, either as a result of cell necrosis or because of inflammatory reaction surrounding and overcoming the incipient 'tumour'. The viruses form a graded series. In a number of the more typical poxes such as vaccinia, the evolution of the lesions takes place over a matter of days. The wart-like lesions of fowl-pox may persist for weeks before they resolve, while those of the rabbit fibroma and the Yaba monkey virus may be present for a period of months. The poxviruses are interesting because, even though they do not give rise to progressive growths, they illustrate the point made in chapter 1 that there is no very sharp line of distinction between those viruses which are oncogenic and others, which perhaps only just fail to qualify.

Little need be said concerning the more typical poxes which run a short course: these nearly all make their attack wholly or largely on superficial epithelial cells; they multiply only in cytoplasm and produce therein characteristic inclusion bodies. Some of these inclusions are micro-colonies of virus particles; others are made of masses of incidentally produced protein material. Mention will be made in chapter 17 of some evidence of possible synergic action between carcinogenic chemicals and the viruses of vaccinia and fowl-pox. This is, however, much less striking than in the case with the fibroma virus and other viruses not in the pox family. There is a report from Poland [209] that vaccinia virus in very small doses can induce transformation of cells in primary cultures of mouse embryos, but it is not stated whether contamination with polyoma virus has been excluded. Instead of progressing towards oncogenicity a poxvirus may go the other way. There are reports [61] of a 'pock-less' rabbit pox which caused acute infection with oedema and diarrhoea and finally death : no pocks were seen. *Molluscum contagiosum* is a chronic skin disease of man caused by a poxvirus. The lesions consist of pearly white nodules about 2 mm. across. They begin after an incubation period of fourteen to fifty days with hyperplasia of epithelial cells: many mitoses may be seen. The lesion finally becomes loculated; its large cells contain the so-called molluscum bodies twenty to thirty microns across : these in turn are full of virus particles closely resembling those of vaccinia (plate 22). The nodules may persist for many months before regressing. The virus has not been transmitted to other species : there is evidence that it will multiply in some cultures of human tissues but it has not been serially propagated [282].

Myxoma and fibroma of rabbits. Five closely related viruses form a subgroup of the poxvirus family. One is the well known myxoma virus which naturally infects *Sylvilagus brasiliensis* rabbits in South America: it causes in them purely local lesions, but a fatal generalized infection is caused in Euopean rabbits (*Oryctolagus*) and the domesticated rabbits derived from them. Next comes Shope's fibroma which again causes only local lesions in its natural hosts cottontail rabbits (*Sylvilagus floridanus*), but unlike myxoma virus only local lesions in *Oryctolagus*: exceptions will be mentioned later. A third virus affects *Sylvilagus bachmani* in California, producing fibromata in them and a fatal disease in domestic rabbits : this is clinically quite unlike myxomatosis [233]. Then there is a virus of the family affecting hares (*Lepus*) in North Italy, Southern France and probably elsewhere. Finally there is a fibroma virus affecting grey squirrels (*Sciurus carolinensis*) in North America and serially transmissible also in woodchucks (*Marmota monax*) [194]. It is serologically related to rabbit fibroma. In suckling squirrels it produces generalized skin nodules and also lung adenomata [192, 196]. All these viruses seem to be transmitted by biting insects, but only mechanically: there is no good evidence of a biological cycle in the insects.

Myxomatosis virus deserves mention only because there is cellular proliferation preceding degenerative changes in the gelatinous swellings which are a feature of the disease: acute inflammation of the eyes and elsewhere is very obvious.

Fibromata caused by Shope's [323] virus come to look much more like neoplastic growths. The very earliest changes after inoculation into skin or testes of rabbits consist of hyperaemia, oedema and infiltration with polymorphonuclear cells. Soon, mononuclear cells increase in numbers and there appear more and more young fibroblasts with many mitoses. One soon sees whorls of spindle-shaped cells resulting from this fibroblastic proliferation and one might suspect that they were sarcomata, except that necrosis and regression begin in domestic rabbits after ten or fifteen days. In cottontails, however, fibromata may persist as long as five or ten months before regressing [193].

Such are the changes caused by the classical virus. A derived strain, however, behaved very differently [20, 27]. The early changes were the same but the early inflammation was immediately followed by the necrotic and regressive changes without any intermediate period of fibroblastic overgrowth. It was suggested that the inflammatory variant killed the cells it attacked while the original virus, being of lesser virulence, was able to stimulate cell-growth at any rate until the body's defences had been mobilized. One recalls the attack of the Rous virus on very young chicks leading to the appearance of haemorrhagic lesions instead of sarcomata.

Results of poor response by the host's defensive mechanisms are revealed in several ways. In immunologically immature cottontail or domestic rabbits a few days old, the virus causes a rapidly fatal disease. Virus is present in the blood and there are generalized lesions [374] including 'tumours' in kidneys and sometimes elsewhere. The lesions show both proliferative and inflammatory features [92]. Defensive responses may be suppressed in adult rabbits in a variety of ways. X-irradiation, cortisone and other immuno-suppressive drugs all delay the regression of the fibromata and allow the development of generalized lesions [65, 159]. Antibody formation may be interfered with. However, Allison and Friedman [10] observed that in newborn rabbits fatal results were due to failure of a cellular response rather than to failure to develop antibodies. The rather similar results following treatment with carcinogenic chemicals will be discussed in chapter 17.

As long ago as 1903, von Dungern and Coca [88] reported the occurrence of sarcomata in hares, serially transplantable in domestic rabbits. The authors considered that the rabbit tumours were still composed of hare cells, but in the light of later knowledge this seems improbable. Metastases were reported but the growths apparently always regressed: at any rate there is no mention that any were fatal. Nothing more was heard of these interesting tumours for more than half a century. Then in 1961 'a nodular skin disease of the hares of the Po valley' in Italy was reported [217]: and a similar disease was noted in the south of France. A virus serologically related to that of Shope's fibroma was isolated, and this was serially transmissible in domestic rabbits. It seems highly probable that the disease reported is the same as von Dungern and Coca's 'hare sarcoma' and that the agent is the old-world representative of the myxoma–fibroma group of poxviruses.

The last poxvirus to be considered is the Yaba-monkey virus. This led to the spontaneous appearance of tumour-like growths, especially on heads and limbs, of rhesus monkeys housed in the open at Yaba near Lagos in Nigeria [33] (plate 21). One baboon was also affected. We do not know the natural host of the virus, which may have been arthropod-borne and have thus infected the captive Asiatic monkeys. Growths were readily produced by subcutaneous or intradermal inoculation of rhesus and other Asiatic macaques. They appeared five days after injection of potent suspensions and grew steadily, reaching a maximum in four to six weeks, after which regression began and was usually complete by the sixth to twelfth week after inoculation. Well-grown lesions were firm, circumscribed, pink nodules, 25 to 46 mm. across and projecting 25 mm. above the surrounding skin [25, 260]. The African monkey *Cercopithecus aethiops* was relatively resistant to inoculation: the lesions produced were relatively flat and soon regressed. No success followed attempts to infect two other African species and the South American *Cebus fatuellus*: nor could animals other than primates be infected. The virus could, however, produce transient lesions in man. Grace *et al.* [137] tested the virus on a few cancer patients and recorded also one accidental laboratory infection in man. Skin nodules appeared after five to seven days, reached 2 cm. in diameter and regressed after three to four weeks.

Connective tissue, rather than epithelia, is attacked. The affected cells in the growths are pleomorphic, often polygonal and transitions between them and fibroblasts are seen. Inclusion bodies lying alongside the nucleus are seen in many cells. When regression begins, mononuclear cells collect in large numbers and are found surrounding large necrotic areas.

Electron microscopy reveals the presence of virus particles almost identical with those of vaccinia; but these have proved in serological tests to be unrelated to other poxviruses. The virus has been successfuly grown in a number of primate tissue cultures, also in the yolk-sac and on the chlorio-allantoic membrane of fertile eggs [346]. In some tissue cultures 'microplaques' of heaped-up cells were seen [372]. It seemed likely from various studies that direct cell-to-cell spread of virus was occurring.

15
Tumours in Frogs and Fishes

The small leopard-frog, *Rana pipiens*, is extremely common in North America and it has been said that in spring one can travel from the north to the Mexican border and never be out of range of its chirping song. In northern Vermont and adjacent parts of Canada there is a high incidence of kidney tumours in the frogs. They are adenocarcinomata covering a range from relatively harmless-looking adenomata to highly invasive cancers: apparently they never regress but go on to kill the frogs. They are usually bilateral and appear to start from multiple foci. Some are 'replica tumours' in which the kidney retains its normal shape but has in fact been wholly replaced by tumour cells. Metastases are uncommon in the field but are often seen when frogs are kept in the laboratory. Eosinophilic intranuclear inclusion bodies of Cowdry's [69] A type may be found in large numbers [289].

There is good evidence that a virus is concerned [221, 222] and a few years ago no one doubted that a virus of the herpes family was the causative agent: this has been called the Lucké virus, after its discoverer. Since then, however, things have got more complicated. It appears that the tumours appear in a certain number of control, uninoculated frogs and that all one can accomplish by injection of virus-containing material is to increase the incidence and accelerate the appearance of the growths. One recalls the effect of Gross' leukaemia virus in accelerating the development of the disease in the susceptible AKR mice. One might hope to obtain clear results and wholly negative controls by using frogs from an area where the disease is not endemic. It appears, however, that leopard-frogs of subspecies from elsewhere in the USA may be insusceptible to the virus. The disease has been recognized now in areas formerly thought to be free, for instance Wisconsin and Minnesota. The possibility of cross-infection in the laboratory may also have confused the issue.

When tumour extracts, filtered, dried or glycerolated, are injected by any route, there is no local change and the frogs remain normal for at least three months. After three months, frogs which are killed have twice as many tumours in their kidneys as have uninoculated controls, while later on there is a three-fold difference. When actual tumour tissue is grafted into normal frogs there is no progressive growth locally but, once again, an increased incidence of kidney tumour some months later: in this instance it may be six times as high as in controls. Perhaps the best evidence for transmission is that tumours transplanted into tails or elsewhere in tadpoles, though never persisting after metamorphosis, lead to appearance of kidney growths very soon after that event, at an age when they are hardly ever seen in nature.

Particular interest has attached to the presence in the tumour of the nuclear inclusions. These are just like those associated with members of the herpes virus family (plate 2). Indeed, electron microscopy reveals that the virus particles are just like those of herpes, having a cubical symmetry and 162 capsomeres (plate 1): like herpes, the virus is ether-sensitive, contains DNA and begins its growth in the cell nucleus. A puzzling fact was that the inclusions were sometimes to be found in the tumours and sometimes not. It has since appeared that this all depends upon the temperature. In spring, when the frogs come out of hibernation, inclusions can be found plentifully: later in the year they are absent. Workers in laboratories kept at 15° C. or higher have reported failure to find inclusions in their frogs. One group of workers [242] studied tumours having the 'summer morphology' with numerous mitoses and no inclusions: from these they could obtain no virus. Yet they did so when the tumours or transplants from them were kept in the cold. While higher temperatures inhibit inclusion formation, they favour growth of the tumours, which appear more frequently in frogs kept at 23–6° C.

There is considerable support for the view that infection may normally pass to tadpoles, virus having been passed into the spawn water in the urine of infected frogs: it may then remain latent perhaps until the frogs are in their third summer or later [289].

The tumours can be grown for a limited period in tissue cultures but inclusions are not formed in the cultures. Evidently one level of virus–cell balance is optimal for inclusion formation and another for tumour development. Several workers have failed to infect cultures of adult frog kidney cells or at least saw no definite cytopathic effects, but no studies are reported with tadpole cells nor when cultures were treated with extracts from inclusion-bearing tumours.

A further complication has been the discovery that frog tumours may contain quite a different virus [142], and it cannot be assumed, just because the Lucké virus gives rise to striking inclusion bodies, that it, and not the other virus, is the causative agent. The various viruses isolated have been given numbers, FV (frog virus) 1, 2, 3, 4, etc., but there is no good evidence that more than two are concerned, the Lucké virus and one other, of which the prototype is FV4. This also is an ether-sensitive, DNA-containing virus, but it is found only in cytoplasm, is larger than the other (120 × 130 nm.) [72] and is morphologically similar to a virus isolated from crane-flies (*Tipula*), though the latter is ether-resistant. The larger frog virus can be cultivated in tissues of various, including mammalian, species. The Lucké virus is, however, the more likely candidate for the role of causative agent of the tumour. Came and Lunger [53] found the cytoplasmic one in only three of thirty-four tumours (8·8 per cent) against thirty-one of thirty-four (91·2 per cent) for the Lucké virus. It has been suggested [361] that the nuclear virus might act as a helper for the cytoplasmic one.

Rose and Rose [294] found that tumour tissue implanted in immature salamanders (*Triturus*) or in adult salamanders during limb regeneration would give rise to osteochondromata.

Toad lymphosarcoma

A lymphosarcoma has been described in South African clawed toads (*Xenopus laevis*) [29, 30]. It was transmitted by means of filtrates to *Xenopus*, frogs (*Rana pipiens*) and newts (*Triturus*).

The tumours frequently metastasized. The virus was ether-sensitive, passed a 100-nm. membrane and apparently passed from one toad to another in water. It is probably a herpes virus like the Lucké virus.

Lymphocystic disease of fish

In this non-fatal disease there are light-coloured wart-like growths of jelly-like consistency on the skin. The growths are due to spectacular enlargement of epithelial cells, whch may show a more than 100,000-fold increase in volume. The lesions eventually regress. The big lymphocystis cells are less commonly found in internal organs. Within the cytoplasm are inclusion bodies containing DNA, as shown by staining with acridine orange or by Feulgen's method: they may be distributed at the periphery of the cell, around which a hyaline membrane is found. The disease is transmissible with filtrates. The virus contains DNA, is minimally sensitive to ether, has an icosahedral form and is about 300 nm. in diameter. It has been suggested that it may be a poxvirus [369] or possibly related to the *Tipula* iridescent virus and the cytoplasmic frog viruses [238].

Lymphocystis disease occurs in fish of several families including flounder, plaice, perch and bluegills, but transmission is not very easy with material from one fish family to those of another; the suggestion has therefore been made that there may be a family of related viruses. There is, however, no serological evidence bearing on this possibility. Outbreaks of the disease occur especially in summer months but the mode of spread is uncertain. A role of parasites has been suspected; on the other hand the lymphocystis cells burst in water and may thus spread the disease.

Other fish diseases

A viral cause has been suspected for several other neoplastic diseases of fish. Virus-like particles have been seen in the lesions of sarcomas in the wall-eye or pike-perch (*Stizostedion*), an epidermal hyperplasia, also in wall-eyes, papillomata in flat-fish and fish-pox: there is, however, no experimental evidence that viruses are the causative agents. More definite evidence concerns a virus causing kidney tumours in an aquarium fish (*Pristella*). This, like the virus of kidney tumours in frogs, gave rise to kidney tumours regardless of the route of injection: secondary growths appeared in other organs later. Four of nine species of 'aquarium fishes' proved susceptible, particularly the guppy (*Lebistes*).

16

Burkitt Tumours

A malignant lymphoma is the commonest form of malignant disease in children in parts of Africa: it is called Burkitt's tumour after the surgeon who first drew attention to it [50]. Certain epidemiological evidence strongly suggests that there might be an insect-borne viral cause. The tumour has therefore been intensively studied in the last decade, since it has seemed that among tumours of man it is perhaps the likeliest to reveal the involvement of a causative virus. The tumours grow very rapidly and involve especially the orbits and jaws, so that the unfortunate sufferers present a terrible appearance with much distortion of the face (plate 23). Other organs may be involved: the ovary is one of these. The disease is, as a rule, rapidly fatal, but spontaneous regressions are occasionally seen: moreover the tumours may regress either temporarily or perhaps permanently as a result of chemotherapy (plate 24).

Epidemiological aspects

Most malignant tumours have their highest incidence either very early or late in life: it is suggested that this is because defensive mechanisms have in one case not fully matured and in the other case are waning. Burkitt's tumour, however, has its peak incidence between six and seven years of age. 50 per cent of a long series of cases occurred between five and nine years and 98 per cent before the age of twenty. Up to the age of six or seven there is a roughly 60 per cent increase in absolute incidence per year. It is suggested by Haddow [157] that there may be a passive immunity of maternal origin protecting very young children. Thereafter they are for a while sheltered at home, but from the age of three begin to move more and more freely in the outside world where they may meet a hypothetical infectious agent.

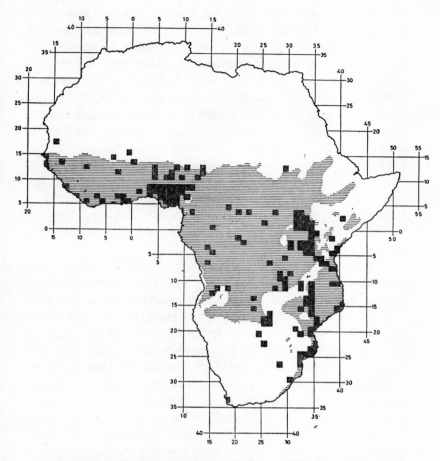

Incidence of Burkitt's tumour in relation to climactic conditions.

The shaded area represents the area in which, on climatological grounds, Burkitt's lymphoma syndrome might be expected to occur.

The black squares show the distribution of the series of cases compiled by Mr Burkitt.

The method here used has been to fill in (in black) any degree-square where the condition has been recorded, irrespective of the number of cases.

It should be remembered that an apparently heavy concentration of cases may simply imply intensive study of the area concerned.

It is the geographical distribution which particularly triggered off the current intensive search for a cause. The vast majority of African cases occur in a wide belt across Africa, as shown in the map [156] (p. 105). This is the region in which the annual rainfall is more than twenty inches and where the mean temperature of the coolest month is less than 60°F. In this area there are many mosquitoes and much mosquito-borne virus disease. In Uganda yellow fever infection is rarely seen at over 5000 ft. altitude, and above this level Burkitt's tumour is very uncommon. This fits in with the 60°F. limiting factor just referred to. Between 60° and 65°F. many viruses cease to develop in mosquito vectors. As to the effect of rainfall, Haddow points out that where the annual precipitation is below twenty inches, many mosquitoes belong to species which rely for survival on drought-resistant eggs: a regular chain of infection would be broken in the temporary absence of adult mosquitoes.

Outside Africa, Burkitt's tumour occurs in New Guinea where climatic conditions are similar [357]. There are, however, parts of Africa, well studied and apparently suitable; yet no Burkitt's tumours are recorded. Still more important is the fact that typical cases of the lymphoma occur from time to time in temperate countries in subjects who have never visited the tropics. The virological evidence to be discussed indicates that these are in all respects like the tropical cases: the hypothetical virus-borne agent is not likely therefore to be the essential one and only cause. An interesting phenomenon in Uganda has been put on record [278] and referred to as epidemic drift: cases beginning at about the same time were shown to live closer together than would be expected on the basis of chance.

These facts of course stimulated several groups of workers to look for an infectious agent, and such agents were duly found. Among the first were the virus of herpes simplex and mycoplasmas. These are known to be present in some normal people, and they can be quickly dismissed as being irrelevant to the problem. Two viruses, however, are of much greater interest: first a herpeslike virus known as the EB virus from the Epstein–Barr cell-line in which it was first recognized [105, 106, 107], and second, a reovirus.

The EB virus

Several workers have succeeded in growing lymphomatous tissue from Burkitt's tumour in culture, and in most of the cell-lines so grown it has been possible to see intranuclear inclusions of Cowdry's A type [69]: these are characteristic particularly of infections by members of the herpes virus group (plate 2). However, it has not been possible as yet to obtain free infectious virus and to infect normal cultures with it: further, there is good immunological evidence that it is not one of the known herpes viruses. Reference has been made in earlier chapters to the virus of Marek's disease and the Lucké frog virus: both of these are so closely cell-associated as not to be readily demonstrated as free infectious agents. The same seems to be true for the EB virus. It has, however, proved possible to infect normal human leucocytes by growing them in culture along with Burkitt cells which have been inactivated by X-rays [169]. Virus is apparently able to pass direct from the tumour cells to the normal cells. The truth of this interpretation is attested by the fact that Burkitt cells from male children have apparently transferred virus to leucocytes from female infants: the sex of infected cells has been ascertained by examining the chromosomes.

The EB virus is present also in certain other tumours, cells of which have been cultivated: nasopharyngeal carcinomas are among these. The virus is also present in some 'normal' cell-lines and in some cases of leukaemia. Nor is it regularly present in Burkitt tumours: there are some cultivated lines of tumour cells from which it is apparently wholly absent.

Several workers have studied immunological aspects of the subject. Old and his co-workers [267] described antibody present in human sera against an antigen present in cultivated Burkitt cells: this was revealed in gel-diffusion tests. Incidence of antibodies was high in African patients with the tumour (31/55 positive), also in people both in Africa and America with carcinoma of the postnasal space (33/39 positive). Only 11 per cent were positive in a total of 258 controls of various categories. An antibody against a Burkitt antigen could be made by immunizing rabbits and was demonstrated by conjugating it with fluorescein and testing against

Burkitt cultures [104]. Klein and his colleagues [200] also used a fluorescent antibody test, employing sera from Burkitt tumour patients and others. Many of the Burkitt patients gave positive tests, especially those reacting well to chemotherapy. Twelve normal Swedes gave negative results. Other workers [131] have found complement-fixing antibodies in 90 per cent of human sera, whether or not they had cancer. They reacted with a Burkitt tumour culture in which EB virus was abundant, not with one in which it was absent. Antibodies were also present in sera of various primates: sera from all chimpanzees and cynomolgus monkeys gave positive results, also some from rhesus and *Cercopithecus*. Sera from species other than primates were all negative.

The whole matter took on a different complexion as a result of discoveries by Dr and Mrs Henle and their colleagues [168]. They were using the fluorescent antibody test in a survey of incidence against EB virus in human sera and a search for conversion from positive to negative. At the same time they were interested in the fact that leucocytes from Burkitt patients would grow out continuously in culture, as those from normal persons would not. White cells and sera from a technician in their laboratory had been tested and had behaved like those of a normal person. She then had an attack of infectious mononucleosis, otherwise known as glandular fever: six rays later her mononuclear blood cells had developed the capacity to grow out in culture and she had now got antibodies against Burkitt antigen. This surprising clue was at once followed up. Fortunately there were available at Yale some sera collected as part of a prospective study of infectious mononucleosis (IM). All thirty-four IM sera turned out to have Burkitt antibodies, as against 24 per cent in controls [259]. Other workers soon confirmed these results and there remains little doubt that the EB virus is in fact the causative agent of IM. It remained undiscovered for so many years largely because of the difficulty in demonstrating free virus, not associated with cells. It is of interest that in IM patients, anti-EB virus antibodies remain high for some time, while the heterophile antibody test, long used in diagnosis, soon becomes negative. It turned out also that leucocytes from IM patients behaved like those of Burkitt patients in growing out well in culture. The fluorescent antibody tests were,

by the way, negative against a line of Burkitt cells lacking EB
virus.

Miscellaneous findings

Before discussing the significance of these discoveries it will be
well to mention some other clues, misleading or otherwise, into the
nature of the Burkitt tumour or the EB virus. Epstein has pointed
out that the EB virus closely resembles the Lucké frog virus in its
unusual association with spindle tubules in the cell and that a
similar virus occurs in tumours in an African amphibian (*Xenopus*)
[30]. Moreover some mosquitoes are known to bite both amphibians and human beings. Epstein [107] has also attempted
transmission of Burkitt material to African monkeys: bone lesions
appeared in two of three *Cercopithecus* surviving for more than
two years. There were cystic destruction of bone and collections
of what were interpreted as being lymphoblastic cells. Discussion
of these findings revealed considerable doubts as to whether the
lesions in these monkeys were neoplastic: it was also maintained
that similar lesions were apt to occur in monkeys kept a long time
in captivity. Another report [336] is that Burkitt material will produce brain lesions when injected into newborn thymectomized
mice and hamsters: the condition was transmissible in series but
EB virus inclusions were not seen in the lesions. Finally, what appeared to be EB virus was detected in cultivated leucocytes of normal chimpanzees [213]: this of course could indicate only that
chimpanzees are subject to infection by a virus related to that of
human IM or had picked up the human infection.

Reoviruses

There is no great significance in the fact that reoviruses have on a
number of occasions been cultivated from Burkitt tumour
material: they apparently occur not uncommonly in animals of
many species, including man. The finding derives its interest
largely from the work of Stanley and his colleagues in Australia on
reovirus infections of mice. They first recovered reovirus type 3,
apparently from a human case, and called it 'hepato-encephalitis
virus' from the effects produced in suckling mice. Most inoculated
mice died, but survivors developed a runting disease from which

virus was no longer recoverable. Spleen cells transferred to genetically similar newborn mice reproduced the runting disease, which the authors explained as an auto-immune reaction induced by the reovirus infection. Then some, though only a few, of the runt mice developed a lymphoma histologically like Burkitt's lymphoma, largely mesenteric in distribution but sometimes affecting the jaws. The lymphomata were transmissible in series: they yielded no virus directly but reovirus was recovered by irradiating tumour cells and growing them on feeder layers of normal mouse cells [335]. There was serological evidence, also, of a relation between the lymphomata and the reovirus [334]. It has, however, been reported that such a lymphoma examined by the electron microscope contains virus particles considerably larger than those of a reovirus [274]. A recent report [36] describes a multifocal malignant lymphoma occurring in one of two rabbits seven months after a series of intravenous injections of reovirus; no reovirus antigen, however, was detected in the tumours.

Interpretation of findings

Are Burkitt's tumours due to the EB virus, to reovirus, to some other virus, or is a virus not concerned at all? Quite obviously, the EB and reoviruses could both be passengers. It has been shown that reovirus can survive in a carrier state in Burkitt cells [219]. There is no evidence supporting the idea that one could act as a helper of the other. The notion that cancer could develop out of an auto-immune disease is not a new one and makes the study of the host-reovirus relationship well worth further study. On the other hand Stanley was studying mice with a graft versus host reaction and since malignancies are known to arise out of such things, the lymphomata may have resulted from the graft versus host reaction as such, irrespective of whether it had a viral cause. The much greater frequency of occurrence of the EB virus entitles it to particular attention. Though occurrence of incidental viruses as passengers in tumours is familiar, it would be odd to find a particular virus occurring so frequently in particular tumours: there could, however, be a type of cell in which the IM virus found it especially easy to settle down in a long-term association. In favour of its causative role is the fact that the IM virus can cause leucocytes to persist for a long time in culture. This is rather a characteristic of malignant cells and it has been suggested that this virus is half-way to an oncogenic virus, causing a self-limited sort of lymphomatosis. In any case one has to explain why Burkitt's tumour occurs very sporadically in temperate countries but is frequent and endemic in some tropical regions. A helper action by an arbovirus has been suggested but confirmatory evidence is lacking. Allison [9], developing an idea put forward by Dalldorf [70], has offered another explanation:

I.M. virus normally produces a self-limiting proliferation of mononuclear cells, but ... if the subject is already reacting to an intense and prolonged antigenic stimulus, there is an increased probability that the proliferative response to the virus will go over to frank malignancy ... Holoendemic malarial infection is an example of such an intense proliferative stimulus ... the distribution of Burkitt lymphoma parallels that of holoendemic malaria.

One might hope that more detailed comparison of incidence of malaria and lymphoma and of the effect of antimalarial measures would soon demonstrate the truth or otherwise of this ingenious suggestion. Meanwhile there are many workers trying to discover which if any of rival hypotheses comes near to the truth, and the answer should not be long in coming.

17

Experiments on Synergism

One of the unanswered questions in cancer research is whether viruses should be regarded merely as one type of carcinogen among many – chemical and physical agents being others: or whether one should regard viruses as being universal continuing causes of neoplastic growth. In the latter case physical or chemical carcinogens could be regarded as activating a virus.

Several workers have carried out experiments designed to throw light on this question, and suggestive results have been obtained involving viruses of several sorts. By way of background one may refer to some old experiments by Goodpasture [135]: he showed that herpes simplex virus would produce lesions on the tarred skins of guinea pigs, though his strain failed to do so in the absence of tar.

The most striking results were obtained by Rous and his colleagues working with Shope's rabbit papilloma. Their work revealed that there could be a synergistic action between chemical carcinogens and viruses. Two types of experiments were carried out. In the first [293], areas of rabbits' skins were scarified and papilloma virus was rubbed in: then the scarified area was covered with dressings containing either the carcinogenic hydrocarbons 20-methylcholanthrene or 9,10-dimethyl-1,2-benzanthracene. Cancers arose from the resulting papillomata much sooner than from other rabbits whose dressings had contained non-carcinogenic substances. In a second type of experiment [191, 300], ears of rabbits were painted with a tar which could elicit in rabbits benign warts but rarely cancer. When warts had appeared papilloma virus was given intravenously. About three weeks later papillomas probably due to the virus appeared, and simultaneously the tar warts 'previously indolent, began to enlarge with great rapidity' and in fact many of them soon declared themselves as invasive carcinomata, appearing much sooner than would have happened from the action of either tar or virus alone. To produce this effect quite vigorous preliminary treatment with tar was necessary: much less drastic tarring served only to localize papilloma to the tarred area when virus was given intravenously: the warts then appearing were ordinary virus warts.

Sarcomata have been induced in fowls by injecting tar or carcinogenic hydrocarbons. Many such tumours have been obtained in this way but most of them have not been propagable in series. A few workers have obtained active filtrates from such tumours [225], but failure to do so has been a much more usual experience. One has to be very cautious in interpreting the positive results: McIntosh's experiments have been especially criticized, and for two reasons: his fowls had a high incidence of leukaemia, and the tumours he obtained mostly appeared at sites other than where the tar was injected. It would be desirable as a precaution to carry out such experiments in a laboratory where known filterable tumours are not present.

I carried out some experiments [21] bearing on this question on pheasants. As mentioned in chapter 6, several filterable fowl tumours were readily transmitted to pheasants, some of them by means of filtrates, and there was thus good evidence that the resulting tumours were composed of pheasant cells. It thus seemed worth while to see how propagable but non-filterable fowl tar tumours would behave in pheasants. Minced tumour of the Sheffield tar sarcoma was injected into the breast muscles of seventeen adult pheasants and some growth occurred in fifteen of them. In most the tumour only grew for about fourteen days, reaching a diameter of 1 to 5 cm., and then regressing. In two pheasants, however, growth continued for several weeks till the breast on one side was enlarged to two or three times its normal size. However, after fifty-four and thirty-six days respectively, regression occurred. It is perhaps worth mentioning that one of these two pheasants had earlier been injected with dried tar-tumour material: no tumour resulted; conceivably it had been rendered tolerant to the tumour cells. The evidence suggested that the tumours in most of the birds were due to surviving fowl sarcoma cells, for the previous injection of minced chicken embryo rendered them resistant rather than tolerant to the tumour injection. It must be mentioned that even in fowls regressions and failures to take were frequent with the Sheffield tumour, and that in one experiment 'takes' were much better in pheasants than in fowls.

The main interest of this work lies in the serological findings. Sera of one of the pheasants which had developed a large tumour contained potent neutralizing antibodies against the Rous virus; so did five of six sera from birds in which tumours had only been palpable for a short time. Experiments of several kinds indicated that these were specific antiviral antibodies. No neutralization of the Rous virus was effected by sera of twenty-one normal adult pheasants. It was concluded that 'the non-filterable Sheffield tar tumour contains a virus which is responsible for calling forth antibodies in inoculated pheasants. The virus must be closely related serologically to that of Rous No. one. It is probably but not certainly responsible for maintaining the malignant properties of the tumour cells.' In the light of recent work, it seems that the caution in the last sentence may have been justified. It seems not unlikely that the Sheffield tumour had in the course of passage through fowls picked up as passenger virus an RAV virus such as was desscribed in chapter 4. Fowls grafted with the Sheffield tumour also develop antibodies to Rous virus: in view of the occurrence of such antibodies in some normal fowls, the result is perhaps even harder to interpret than in the case of the pheasants. However, sera from some primary tumours in fowls which Dr P. R. Peacock kindly allowed me to bleed had in many cases no anti-Rous antibodies. Moreover Gusev [149] showed that while all Rous sarcomata showed cross-reactions in gel-diffusion tests, chemically induced tumours did not react with the anti-Rous sera. In interpreting such negative findings it must be remembered that there are now known to be fowl-tumour viruses serologically distinct from those studied earlier.

The rabbit fibroma described in chapter 14 is a growth which commonly regresses and is not admitted by pathologists generally to be a 'true tumour'. Its behaviour is, however, profoundly modified by tar-injection [2]. Rabbits were injected intramuscularly with a tar known to be carcinogenic and with dilutions of fibroma virus (OA strain) intradermally. The resulting fibroma lesions regressed by the end of a month in control rabbits, while those in the tarred animals persisted for two to four months. Histologically the growths in tarred animals revealed more tightly packed cells, which at times were arranged very irregularly: the picture resembled that seen in the growths in cottontails: these are usually more chronic than in tame rabbits. When fibroma virus was given intravenously to tarred rabbits, the virus localized, as might be expected, at the site of the intramuscular tar injections. The rabbits also showed evidence of generalized fibromatosis: nodules appeared in various places, especially subcutaneously, but some were attached to bone and some appeared at mucocutaneous junctions. Most appeared within ten days of the virus injection and they usually persisted for some time, though at times they regressed while new ones were still appearing. In contrast to ordinary fibroma lesions, there was little cell reaction around them. Virus of the ordinary kind was readily recoverable from them. Some of the animals showed emaciation and died within a month: in others the course was much slower while many eventually recovered completely.

A long course of tarring was not necessary to achieve these results: one intramuscular tar injection four or five days before the virus injection was as good as several. Several carcinogenic hydrocarbons, particularly 3,4-benzpyrene and methylcholanthrene, gave similar results, though they were less potent than tar. Noncarcinogenic hydrocarbons and several irritant substances were ineffective. It is not clear how the carcinogens acted: they had no apparent effect on the development of antibodies against the virus. The paper adds, however, 'one is tempted to believe that there may be some mechanism for the intracellular restraint of a parasitic virus and it may well be such a mechanism, if it exists, which is damaged by a toxic agent in tar'. More than twenty years later it was shown that carcinogens inhibit the production of interferon (see p. 129).

In one of the virus-infected rabbits under investigation, a sarcoma appeared at the site of the tar injection in the thigh [23]. This animal had received several injections and paintings of tar over a period of four months before it was given virus. A firm swelling 70 × 50 × 30 mm. appeared: after three months it had become much smaller but thereafter growth was resumed. A biopsy revealed changes suggesting sarcoma: no virus was recovered. After this the tumour grew more rapidly and the rabbit had to be killed six months after the virus injection. There was growth in a mass of lymph-nodes at the bifurcation of the aorta. Transplantation was attempted and was possible only by making passages a few days before regression was likely to set in. After the fourth passage, however, a progressive sarcoma was obtained and this was maintained without difficulty by passage of minced tumour. It was noted that 'it was necessary to expend some time with the scissors to obtain a mince which could be forced through the needle of a tumour-syringe'. Despite the use of various expedients, no virus was obtained from these tumours, and tumour-bearing rabbits were susceptible to inoculation with fibroma virus: moreover, the tumour could be readily transplanted into fibroma-immune animals. In two rabbits in which the tumour had completely regressed, intravenous injection of fibroma virus led to resumption of growth of the sarcomata. This results recalls some of those which Rous and Kidd reported on the effects of giving papilloma virus to rabbits with tar-warts on their ears.

A second sarcoma was obtained by Foulds and Gye, by a similar combination of treatment by tar and fibroma virus; [24] this, however, could not be serially transplanted. It seems unlikely that these two tumours were caused by tar alone: there is a report in the literature of production of a sarcoma in a rabbit by injecting 3,4-benzpyrene intramuscularly [203], yet other workers have failed to produce such tumours in rabbits. It is of some interest that infection by the inflammatory (IA) variant of fibroma virus (see p. 96) was in no way enhanced by treatment with tar.

More recently Kato and his colleagues [187] have obtained fatal fibrosarcomata in rabbits by combined treatment with radioactive cobalt and prednisolone.

Radiation and virus in murine leukaemia

X-irradiation can lead to leukaemia in mice of low-leukaemia lines and from such tumours a transmissible leukaemogenic virus can be isolated. The story is a complicated one, being unravelled by what Kaplan [186] terms 'a twenty-five-year journey through the uncharted twists and turns of research'. It was at first supposed that these leukaemias were the consequence of the mutagenic effects of X-rays, but the facts now make it clear that nothing as simple as routine mutation is concerned. The first fact contradicting that view is that a dose of radiation given in fractions at intervals of a few days is much more effective than if it is given all at once. It appears that presence of the thymus is necessary, since previous thymectomy prevents the occurrence of radiation leukaemia: probably the right target-cells for virus attack are present especially in the thymus. To produce leukaemia, irradiation of both thymus and bone-marrow is essential and leukaemia can be prevented by giving injections into irradiated hosts of isologous marrow cells from non-irradiated mice. It is thought that presence of intact marrow provides protection against leukaemia. The most striking experiment was this: mice were thymectomized and then irradiated: the thymectomy should protect them against leukaemia. Some received grafts of isologous thymus subcutaneously and tumours appeared in these grafts. There was evidence that they arose in the cells of those grafts which had never been irradiated themselves but were growing in the environment of an irradiated mouse.

Lieberman and Kaplan [220] showed that leukaemia viruses could be recovered from the radiation-induced lymphomas, though at first these were only active in low dilutions when given intraperitoneally. It was found later that if filtrates were injected directly into thymus grafts placed under the renal capsule, results were far better. It appeared from electron-micrographs and other studies that the agents obtained from the radiation growths were of essentially the same nature as other murine leukaemic viruses. There was evidence of vertical transmission and of transfer to rats as well as mice.

Lieberman and Kaplan's work was confirmed by Gross, and in

other laboratories it was shown that other carcinogenic agents were able, like X-rays, to cause leukaemias from which a virus was obtainable. Among these were carcinogenic hydrocarbons, urethane and 4-nitroquinoline. Kaplan has marshalled reasons for believing that the viruses so recovered are the cause of the continuing lymphomatous proliferation and are not mere 'passenger viruses'. He suggests that the well-studied 'virulent' Friend, Moloney and Rauscher viruses are not representative of leukaemia viruses as they occur in nature. Rather they have had their properties modified by their opportunities for exuberant growth in the unnatural environment of propagable tumours: for it is from these that they have been obtained. The vertically-transmitted 'temperate' viruses may well represent the normal state of affairs: they may be almost ubiquitous viruses, existing in mice throughout their lives, neither producing leukaemia nor harming them in any other way in the absence of very infrequent activating factors.

It may be mentioned also that there have been several reports suggesting synergistic action between chemical carcinogens and the mouse tumour virus considered in chapter 7. Tumour development in mice infected with that virus may be increased if the mice are treated with a carcinogen, or the virus, hitherto undetected, may be activated [references in Blair, 43]. Similar results have been recorded with polyoma [309].

Carcinogens and poxviruses

Duran-Reynals with Bryan [94] studied a breed of hens which had a latent infection with fowl-pox virus. They found that painting the skin with a solution of methylcholanthrene first activated that latent infection and then led to the appearance of papillomas and cancer. The fowl-pox probably played no role in causing these since they could equally well be brought forth in other breeds of hens which were not carrying fowl-pox. It was found that if adults of these breeds were infected with fowl-pox, virus was quickly eliminated. If, however, fifteen-day-old embryos were infected via the chorio-allantoic membrane, virus, though otherwise recoverable for only fifteen days after hatching, could be activated every time, if birds were painted with methylcholanthrene four months later.

Duran-Reynals [93] then studied vaccinia virus in the skins of mice and found that lesions were enhanced in mice injected with cortisone. When mice were tarred over a period of time, then injected with cortisone and finally with vaccinia, the vaccinial lesions which appeared duly regressed, leaving a scar. Papillomata and other overgrowths appeared where the skin had been tarred but especially in the sites where the vaccinia had been injected into cortisone-treated mice: no virus was recoverable from these. The effect of the virus may have been that of a promoter, as described by Rous but, says Duran-Reynals, 'one may be tempted to envisage the possibility that a non-infective component of the virus is involved in the development of the neoplasms.'

Nature of the synergism

This chapter has recorded a number of examples in which neoplasms have apparently been produced by the combined action of viruses and carcinogenic agents, either chemical or physical. It by no means follows, however, that the mechanism is the same in each case. Papilloma virus drives on tar-warts in rabbits to more active growth: conversely when dressings containing carcinogens were applied to virus warts, cancers appeared much more quickly than happened when other kinds of dressings were used. Viruses have at times, but more often not, been recovered from fowls treated with tar or carcinogenic hydrocarbons: or else serological evidence has been obtained that viruses were active in these tumours. Tar and carcinogens are clearly able to reduce the resistance of rabbits to fibroma virus and occasionally true neoplasms have resulted. There is evidence that carcinogens can activate latent infections with poxviruses. All these suggestive results are made more significant by the very definite effects of X-radiation on mice: here there is clear evidence that activation of a latent virus by a physical carcinogen is related to the appearance of a malignant disease, leukaemia.

How then do the carcinogens act? They are known to be mutagenic, but Kaplan's results with X-rays and leukaemia viruses render it unlikely that mutagenesis is concerned in that phenomenon. They have a depressing effect on antibody production, but this doesn't seem to apply in the case of the activation of fibroma

E

virus. Their other actions are many and various but one cannot see in what way they could help to determine the onset of malignancy. One action is, however, worth more attention. The de Maeyers [79] have shown that carcinogenic hydrocarbons inhibit interferon production and it is known that oncogenic viruses, like most other viruses, are susceptible to interferon. In rat and mouse tissue cultures methylcholanthrene and other compounds significantly reduced interferon production, while other components, chemically related to these but non-carcinogenic, failed to do so. An easy way of comparing the activity of these compounds was to pretreat with them monolayers of cells growing under an agar overlay. A suitably diluted virus such as Semliki forest virus was added and the resulting plaques observed. If interferon formation was suppressed, the virus could extend its activities further before it was checked by interferon formation, and so the plaques were larger than in controls. The effect was not seen in cultures of primate cells: this is not surprising since primates are relatively insusceptible to the carcinogenic effects of these hydrocarbons.

The substances tested are structurally related to steroids, some of which, like cortisone, can inhibit interferon production. Tests were therefore made on a number of other carcinogens such as 4-nitroquinoline-O-oxide, and similar results were obtained: again non-carcinogenic analogues were ineffective. Experiments were also carried out in vivo. The carcinogen urethane was given intraperitoneally to young mice in which interferon production had been induced by giving Newcastle disease (NDV) or Sindbis virus: there was a dramatic though transient drop in the level of circulating interferon. X-irradiation of mice had a depressing effect on the interferon resulting from injection of NDV, less so on that induced by Sindbis virus. This may be explicable on the basis that interferon is made by different cells in response to infection by these two viruses and that in the case of the Sindbis virus the cells are less radio-sensitive.

These experiments suggest that the enhancing effect of carcinogens on virus-caused tumours may, in at least some instances, be due to an effect on interferon production. The de Maeyers suggest that carcinogens may have other, direct, effects on cells, causing cancer in the absence of any participation by a virus: it is admitted that evidence for this is lacking. It could be that an effect on a hitherto undetected virus is concerned: or that the carcinogens are inhibiting some undescribed repressor substances: or that they are depressing an immunological mechanism which normally avails to prevent the acceptance of transformed and potentially malignant cells.

18
Viral Oncolysis

Many viruses multiplying in cells can kill them: some grow particularly well in cancer cells and viruses introduced into a host may localize in cancer cells. The question has naturally arisen as to whether viruses may not be used to cause destruction of tumours. Some kinds of irradiation under certain conditions can cause cancer: under other conditions they can cure. Could the same be true of virus infections? This possibility is the basis of the subject of tumour destruction or oncolysis by viruses.

Viruses have been shown to be capable of causing regressions in transplantable tumours in experimental animals. Such observations have limited significance, for a tumour growing in a genetically foreign host is at a disadvantage anyway and it may not take much to tilt the balance in favour of the host. Nevertheless, some facts of interest emerged from early work on viruses growing in transplantable tumours. This was reviewed by Alice Moore [247] and references to particular papers will be found in that review. It is clear that some viruses cause tumour necrosis and regression, even though there is no generalized illness in the injected animal. Viruses such as influenza A and Newcastle disease virus, when mixed with suspensions of cells of an ascites tumour in mice, will inhibit its growth even though the viruses show no evidence of multiplying themselves. This, however, is an exceptional state of affairs. On the whole, and apart from reasons to be mentioned shortly, arboviruses, and especially those of Casals' B group [56], have given the best results [207]. Against several mouse tumours and also against the RPL 12 strain of fowl leukosis, the West Nile and tick-borne encephalitis viruses have proved very destructive. Yet even within the B group of arboviruses there are remarkable differences. Against three mouse tumours the West Nile virus was effective, as were three other related viruses: yet another, that of Japanese B encephalitis, increased to high titres in the tumour but caused no oncolysis. The tick-borne virus, earlier known as Russian spring–summer encephalitis, was very destructive of a mouse sarcoma. It was also, unfortunately, lethal for most mice, but in a strain of mice resistant to its lethal effects, it was equally good as an oncolytic agent.

Besides the varying behaviour of related viruses, there is unpredictable resistance to the oncolytic effects of any particular virus on the part of different tumours. Some carcinomata and some sarcomata are susceptible, some not. At times a virus has been 'trained' to become oncolytic for a particular tumour by means of serial passages in that tumour. In general, injected viruses have proved to have little effect on the progress of mouse leukaemias, though there may sometimes have been a little inhibition as judged by the sizes of livers and spleens in inoculated and control mice.

From all this work it would clearly be impossible to predict what effect viruses would have on human cancer cells: so, with an eye on possible practical application to human cancer, work has been concentrated on the effects of viruses in malignant cells of human origin. A number of strains of such cells are being propagated in laboratories all over the world: the HeLa and HEp2 lines are among the best known. Before tests have been made in human beings with cancer, as much as possible has been learnt by testing potential oncolytic viruses against cancer-cell lines. Four methods have been used: viruses have been tested for their effects on such cells in tissue culture, on cells growing on the chorio-allantoic membranes of fertile eggs, in the cheek-pouches of hamsters [371] or in rats. It has proved possible to maintain human cancer cells in rats for considerable periods, if the rats are first treated by irradiation or with cortisone to suppress their immune defences against foreign cells. With the help of such techniques it has proved possible to carry out screening tests to see which viruses would be likely to make the best oncolytic agents.

It has been agreed that the most promising viruses would be exotic ones, that is viruses from distant parts of the world against which patients would be unlikely to have pre-existing antibodies. Viruses of most families have a world-wide distribution: exceptions are, however, numerous among the arthropod-borne viruses or arboviruses. Accordingly, it is among the arboviruses that the ideal oncolytic virus has particularly been sought. An obvious requisite is that the chosen virus should not be in itself more than mildly pathogenic.

Much of the work in this field has been carried out by Drs Chester Southam and Alice Moore at the Sloane–Kettering institute in New York [333]. They tested eleven arboviruses and three others against human cancer-cell lines and some other cells. Bunyamwera virus was very destructive for all the cells tested, most others rather less so or only against some of the cell lines. Growth curves were plotted for all the viruses in all the cell lines and it was seen that virus growth and destructive effect did not always run parallel. Tests were next made on the power of the viruses to inhibit growth of one line of tumour cell, HEp3, growing in eggs. Effects were gauged by the suppression of ability of virus-treated cells to grow when passed to further eggs or to cortisone-treated rats. The viruses had roughly but not precisely the same efficiency as when noted in tissue cultures.

In direct tests in rats it was found best to do similar bioassays by passage to further rats, rather than relying on any direct effect on the size of the tumours in the original rats. The viruses to come out best from such a trial run were the Bunyamwera and Egypt 101 virus. The latter is a strain of West Nile virus, a mosquito-borne arbovirus. Taking all its properties into account, this West Nile virus was judged to be the most promising for tests in man. In view of the doubt as to the value of such tests, it was decided to employ them only in patients with an otherwise hopeless prognosis. Eighty-four patients so tested lived long enough to permit evaluation of the results, which are set out in table 2. Virus was given intramuscularly and patients' blood was taken daily for injection into mice to see whether viraemia developed. Biopsies were also carried out.

Ninety per cent of the patients developed an active infection as shown by the occurrence of viraemia over two or three days. Nine of them (11 per cent) had symptoms of encephalitis, severe in two instances. The column in the table marked 'selection' indicates that in these patients more virus was present in the tumour tissue taken at biopsy than in the blood or other tissues. Tumour inhibition was assessed by measurement of tumour size when this was possible or by X-ray evidence.

The results were not encouraging. Only 8 per cent of patients showed any evidence of tumour regression and this improvement was not maintained. The occurrence of encephalitis after injection of a reputedly harmless, or nearly harmless, virus was disquieting and may well have been due to the fact that immunological defences may be diminished in terminal cancer patients. The en-

Table 2. *Effect of West Nile Virus on Growth of Cancer in Man*

Type of cancer	Localization			Inhibition of tumour		
	No	Yes	Selection (see text)	No	?	Yes
Carcinomas						
Epidermoid	3	5	5	14	1	0
Gastro-intestinal	0	14	5	24	5	3
Other	1	4	1	8	0	0
Sarcomas						
Reticulum-cell	0	5	1	2	2	3
Other	1	8	2	8	2	0
Total	5	36	14	56	10	6
Per cent	10	65	25	78	14	8

Modified from Moore [247].

cephalitic symptoms occurred mainly in patients with tumours involving the lymphatic system such as leukaemia or reticular-cell sarcomas.

Results of other workers have been no more promising. Adenoviruses tested against carcinoma of the uterine cervix led apparently to some tumour necrosis but to no permanent improvement [331]. An obstacle in the way of success is that treated patients soon develop antibodies to the injected virus, so that it can no longer be effective. A theoretical possibility is to have available a battery of oncolytic viruses and to use them one after another without giving the tumour cells any respite. In view of the varying effects of viruses on different tumours, not even this approach seems very hopeful, and one cannot claim that prospects of practical usefulness of viral oncolysis are very great.

19
More about Tumour Immunity

Cancer, as is well known, is a disease especially of older people and animals generally. It can be argued that because it attacks mainly those beyond the child-bearing age, evolution by natural selection has been relatively powerless to eliminate it. For many years it was supposed that the greater incidence in old age could be accounted for by the need for specific carcinogenic stimuli to operate over a very long time and by the very slow evolution of most tumours in their early stages. Recently attention has tended to switch to study of immunological aspects. It was pointed out in chapter 12 that immunity to virus tumours depended on cellular rather than humoral factors, and this is doubtless true of tumours in general.

Immunological surveillance

The body does not react against antigens which it recognizes as 'self', but there is increasing evidence that many kinds of neoplastic cells are antigenically different from normal cells and do, therefore, elicit a response. The reaction is akin to that concerned in the rejection of grafts of genetically dissimilar tissues. Burnet [52] has postulated that there exists an 'immunological surveillance mechanism' with the function of eliminating clones of its own cells which do not conform. Tumour cells with strange antigens on their surfaces would fall into this category. Burnet suggests that this may represent the most primitive kind of immunological reaction, having been developed as soon as organisms began to be multicellular.

Klein [199] doubts whether such an immunological mechanism

is adequate and considers that another kind of surveillance, a non-immunological one, may supplement it: this would have to be effected by neighbouring cells actually in contact with a rebellious non-conforming neighbour. Possibly a mechanism may have arisen or been perfected from one directed against parasites: against these, especially larger parasites, a cell-mediated defence is often predominant. The effective cell is generally the lymphocyte which is mobile and can seek out the foreigner, whether of endogenous or exogenous origin, and destroy it. There might be an actual killing or merely an ability to inhibit multiplication, which would amount in practice to the same thing. Klein [199] has discussed at length the possible ways in which all this might be brought about.

There is evidence that humoral mechanisms may also come into play and this is particularly the case with leukaemias, the cells of which are susceptible to attack by sera with specific cytotoxic properties. In the case of the Moloney mouse lymphoma, there is variation in the amount of antigen on the surface of cells: those with higher concentration of antigen are most sensitive to attack.

Failure of surveillance

So much for why we don't get cancer. Fortunately, through one mechanism or another, most of us avoid it for most of our lives; so the defence is evidently effective. Equally clearly, it is not always so, and we must consider why it breaks down. Current opinion considers that this happens when the immune response fails. This, like so many undesirable things, may happen as we grow older. It is on record [171] that patients in the late stages of cancer fail to reject homografts, though other equally debilitated patients can do so (see p. 125). Leaving aside the older people, we find that cancers, especially leukaemias, are commoner in small children than in older ones and young adults, and it is at the beginning of life that cellular immunological responses are poor, as they are relatively slow to develop (see p. 83). There is also the special case of the vertically transmitted viruses of mice; in these instances infection may occur so early that the host has not developed the ability to recognize the virus as 'non-self' and so immunological tolerance results.

Naturally occurring tumours are never known to lose their novel antigen altogether, but these may be much diminished. It was mentioned in chapter 12 that loss of transplantation antigen by an SV 40 tumour was associated with ability to metastasize [77]. It has also been suggested that clones of non-conforming cells which differ antigenically only very slightly from normal are more likely to evade the body's defences. Such clones as these or others which can grow unusually quickly may 'sneak through' the defences and reach an irreversible size before these have been adequately mobilized [199]. Escape also from non-immunological control is possible, if a focus of sufficient size can be created. This possibility was discussed in chapter 11 in relation to the ability of normal cells to restore the property of contact inhibition to transformed cells. A phenomenon possibly related to this was described by Henry Harris and co-workers [160]. Cells of each of three different mouse cancers were fused, with the help of Sendai virus, with those of a normal mouse fibroblast line. Means were available for selecting the hybrid cells, which proved to contain chromosome markers characteristic of both parents. In all three instances the hybrid cells had lost their malignant characters, as shown by the results of injection into suitable mice.

It should be noted, however, that Defendi and his colleagues obtained a contrary result: hybrid cells produced by fusing normal mouse cells with others transformed by polyoma were more oncogenic than the original transformed cells [75]. They suggest that fusion of tumour cells with adjacent normal ones might be concerned in a tumour's invasiveness. The contrast with the findings of Stoker and Harris suggests that the situation is complex and that a shift in the balance of power may determine the outcome.

Role of cell-mediated immunity

A puzzling finding has been that lymphocytes from immune animals may be able to suppress colony formation by tumour cells *in vitro* yet be powerless to check tumour growth *in vivo*. The Hellströms and their colleagues [167] found that if the serum of mice with progressively growing mouse sarcoma (M) tumours (see p. 55) was added to tumour cells *in vitro* before addition of the lymphocytes, their inhibiting effect was abrogated. Sera of mice with regressed tumours had no such effect. Similar results were obtained in the case of rabbit papilloma and mouse-mammary cancer: also with some human tumours, using lymphocytes from the patients' blood. In the last tests there was some crossing of inhibiting powers of sera between several cancers of the colon but not between tumours of colon and some other organs. The results recall the enhancing effect of some antibodies, particularly weak ones, on transplantability of tumour cells. Enhancement, instead of the suppression one might expect, may be due to blocking of receptor sites on the tumour cell's surface, so that the lymphocytes cannot get at it.

The importance of the cell-mediated defence mechanism against cancer has important implications in the currently popular field of organ transplantation. Success here depends not only on the surgeon's skill but on the suppression of the tendency to reject cells or tissues of a genetically foreign host. Earlier use of immunosuppressive drugs was followed only too often by activation of infections, particularly those caused by the cytomegalic inclusion virus, a member of the herpes virus family. Later it was found possible to inhibit more specifically the cellular and not the humoral mechanisms: antilymphocytic serum proved particularly valuable for this purpose. Injection of such serum has been found to increase the susceptibility of infant mice to polyoma [11]. Workers trying to infect mice with human leprosy bacilli could only achieve their aim by removing their thymus glands and treating them with antilymphocytic serum [127]; in one laboratory, all the mice unexpectedly developed tumours due to polyoma virus which was present in the environment. It was accordingly not difficult to forecast that recipients of grafts of kidneys or other organs treated with antilymphocytic serum would suffer abnormal risk of developing cancer. In fact, a number of such patients have developed tumours – apparently lymphomata rather than other tumours [12, 14].

Role of interferon

A defence mechanism of quite different nature depends upon the activity of interferon. This is a protein having activity against viruses of nearly all kinds, formed in cells as a result of stimulus especially by dead or damaged virus. It inhibits the activity of viruses in the cell, and not only their ability to multiply but those processes which lead to transformation and cancer. In chapter 17 it was pointed out that certain carcinogenic hydrocarbons inhibited the ability of cells to produce interferon and it was suggested that this was one possible way in which to explain the synergistic action of chemicals and viruses in the production of cancer. When given at the right time interferon could inhibit the transformation of a strain of mouse cells by SV 40 [359]. It was also effective in suppressing the activity of Friend leukaemia virus in mice [144]. Against acute virus infections interferon has to be given before virus infection and is useless later. Against Friend virus, on the other hand, it was unnecessary to give it beforehand but treatment had to be continued after infection for some time: possibly the disease is kept going by successive cycles of virus multiplication; in a subacute or chronic infection its usefulness may differ from that in one which is acute.

It appears that a potent stimulant to interferon production is a two-stranded RNA. A synthetic substance with similar properties is polyinosinic-polycytidylic acid, or poly I-poly C. This substance was injected into mice two days after implantation of tumours of several types. It led to decreased growth of the tumour, increased survival and sometimes to tumour regression [218]. None of the tumours in this experiment was known to be virus-caused, and the interpretation of the result is still obscure. It is by no means certain that the beneficial effects were due to mobilization of interferon.

Common antigens and specific ones

The final topic in this immunological chapter is one with important bearing on the likelihood that viruses are concerned in cancers generally and not only in some 'freak' tumours of birds and rodents. As already mentioned, tumours caused by one virus, whatever its location or histological character, usually share common tumour antigens, in particular transplantation antigens. This seems not to be so with chemically induced tumours. The cancers in mice caused by chemical carcinogens have different surface antigens: and, not only that, each single tumour caused by one chemical, methylcholanthrene, even on the same mouse, has a different antigen. If this is a valid difference between virus tumours and chemical tumours, it affords good reason to doubt the significance of the synergism discussed in chapter 17 and to believe that the differences between the tumours caused by various classes of oncogenic agents are fundamental.

The matter is, however, not straightforward. There are some types of human tumours which do share common antigens, for instance some of those affecting the colon and some derived from primitive nerve cells (neuroblastomas). Further, it can be shown by more refined methods that not all polyoma tumours are antigenically identical [179]. In a valuable review of the subject [266] Old and Boyse suggest that there may be antigens with group relations as well as more specific ones. If chemicals do act, let us say in human cancers, by activating a virus, we cannot test for possible virus-induced group antigens because we do not know what virus could be concerned. These authors have in fact found that most mice of one strain with tumours induced by methylcholanthrene do develop antibodies against the group antigen of Gross' leukaemia virus. There is evidence also that there may be highly specific as well as common tumour antigens in various breast tumours caused by the mammary-tumour virus of mice [363, 364].

20

Unanswered Questions

Before coming to grips with really fundamental questions, this chapter will touch upon some others which, though on the fringe of the subject, are irritating because we cannot answer them.

Questions concerning some RNA viruses

Despite the enormous amount of work which has been carried out on fowl tumours, almost no attention has been paid to the remarkable fact that filterable oncogenic agents have been found frequently in fowls but in no other bird species. From analogy with other kinds of virus it seems highly improbable that only one kind of bird is liable to infections of this kind. It is true that domestic fowls have been subject to genetic manipulation by breeders as no other bird has been : yet one might expect that something similar would have turned up in ducks, canaries or budgerigars, species which have been domesticated for many years.

One approach would be to look for specific antisera in the sera of other birds, and such a search has been carried out in East Africa. There H. R. Morgan [251] did find antibodies against viruses of the A leukosis group (see p. 30) in sera of wild ducks, francolins, guinea-fowl, bustards and ostriches. They were present also, as one might expect, in sera of domestic fowls, but there was no likelihood of contact between these and the wild birds. In pheasants and other domesticated game birds in the USA no antibodies were found [285]. I also [21] failed to find antibodies in pheasants in Britain. Since the fowl-tumour viruses are not all alike antigenically, it would of course be desirable to make tests against all available serotypes. It is of course possible that there may in other birds be related viruses which are serologically unlike those of the fowl.

Another problem concerns the relationship of the oncogenic viruses of fowls, rodents and other species to other RNA-containing viruses. Several workers have suggested that there may exist a natural taxonomic group of oncogenic RNA-viruses, including those of fowls and rodents. The name leukoviruses has been proposed [111]. Certainly these have much in common, both in their chemical and physical properties and in their biological behaviour, as earlier chapters have made clear. Two points should, however, be borne in mind. They are not necessarily but only potentially oncogenic viruses. Many or most of them seem to exist ordinarily as inapparent infections. Appearance of spontaneous tumours is a relatively uncommon result of infection, though it may be frequent in inbred or otherwise artificially treated strains. Then, again, we do not know enough about their morphology to be able to state that they differ greatly from viruses which are never known to cause tumours. There are many enveloped RNA-viruses, such as the true myxoviruses and the paramyxoviruses of which the morphology is well understood: but there are even more, including most of the arthropod-borne viruses, concerning which we are comparatively ignorant. The occurrence of oncogenic powers in one or more members of nearly all the known virus groups should warn us against using this potentiality as a taxonomic character.

Canine venereal sarcoma

One of the commonest malignant tumours among dogs has the histological character of a sarcoma and is transmitted venereally. It is commonly fatal but may regress. Elsewhere in the animal kingdom natural transplantation of malignant cells from one individual to another is almost unknown: this would be expected, since animals outside laboratories are genetically very heterogeneous.

Naturally, many workers have wondered whether this tumour may not be, in truth, virus-induced. There are viruses, particularly those in the herpes virus group such as that of Marek's disease, so closely cell-associated that a filterable agent has been hard to demonstrate. One might hope to settle the matter by seeing whether the tumours all had the chromosome pattern of the same sex. If the tumours were due to an infectious virus, the tumour cells in a bitch would always have the characters of the female cell. Unfortunately this approach is not possible, for the chromosomes in all the tumours are highly abnormal and are alike in those from all parts of the world [31, 358]. A single report of transmission by means of filtrates to newborn beagle puppies [185] has not been confirmed. Nor can one place too much emphasis on a report that herpes-type inclusions have been seen: for there is a herpes virus infecting dogs, which may have been picked up as has that of herpes simplex in Burkitt tumours. Until there is more evidence, therefore, one has to accept this tumour as being a unique, cell-transmitted, growth.

Possibly, however, this state of affairs is not unique. A contagious reticular-cell sarcoma of the hamster has been described: growths were mainly in the head, neck or larynx. A remarkable and constant chromosome pattern was seen in tumour cells in either sex and it was believed that spread occurred through cell implantation [68].

We come inevitably to discuss the question of whether viruses cause cancer in man. We have already dealt with Burkitt's tumour and the strong possibility that a herpesvirus is concerned. Another herpesvirus comes into the picture in relation to cancer of the cervix uteri in man.

Herpes virus and cervical cancer

It has been reported lately from several laboratories that strains of herpes simplex virus from the genital tract are distinct serologically from those from around the mouth and face. There are other differences between the viruses from the two sites: the genital ones have been referred to as type 2. Nahmias and his colleagues [255, 256] have pointed out that women with superficial genital herpetic lesions commonly have evidence that the neck of the uterus is infected also. They were led from this observation to consider that herpetic infection might be concerned in cancer of the uterine cervix. They pointed out that the epidemiology of cervical cancer has the stamp of a venereal disease, as has that of genital herpes. Cervical cancer is almost unknown in virgins and nuns but is frequent in promiscuous women. 79 per cent of women with cervical cancer had serological evidence of previous infection with type 2 herpes. Moreover 58 of 245 women with genital herpes infection showed in biopsy specimens from the cervix changes which might be regarded as potentially malignant, and in fourteen cases the changes were definitely cancerous. These suggestive findings have been confirmed in other laboratories. No doubt further immunological and other studies will soon reveal how close is the connection between the herpes 2 infection and the subsequent cancers; at present there is no evidence of a causal relationship.

One other human cancer with a possibly viral cause must be mentioned here. Finkel and colleagues [117] observed osteosarcomas in a small percentage of hamsters inoculated with filtrates from a human osteosarcoma. It must be noted, however, that a filterable osteosarcoma of mice was already under study in their laboratory [116], so that confirmation from other laboratories must be awaited. There is, however, suggestive supporting evidence [252]. Studies with fluorescent antibodies revealed that patients with osteosarcomas had a 100 per cent incidence of reactions with a common osteosarcoma antigen. Contacts with such patients were 85–91 per cent, other people only 29 per cent positive. The result suggests contact with an agent producing unrecognized disease in many, osteosarcoma in a few.

Viruses in human cancers generally

Despite these findings, there is no doubt that as regards the generality of cancers in man, and indeed in other mammals, there is no direct evidence that viruses are concerned. Many arguments can be put forward as to why viruses causing human cancers may not be demonstrable [248]. First and most obviously, it may be because they are not concerned. There are, however, many difficulties in the way of proving their relevance if they *are* there. We cannot, for ethical reasons, test, as we can with fowls and mice, if filtrates of tumour will reproduce the disease. We may well find, as we do in many tumours in mice, hamsters and other species, that infectious virus has disappeared from the growths which it undoubtedly originated. Our hypothetical virus may well be a defec-

F

tive one and we probably would not know how to complement and cultivate it.

Several constructive approaches are, nevertheless, possible. Recent work on virus morphology has made it possible to recognize virus particles when we see them, particularly those with a definite structure – an icosahedral capsid, a helical nucleoid or a surface covered with regularly spaced spikes. There may be difficulties: mycoplasmas have in the past been confused with leukaemia viruses in mice. If any human cancers are virus-caused the leukaemias of childhood are as likely candidates as any. Discovery of leukaemia viruses in mice has been followed by the revelation, with increasing difficulty, of viruses in the leukaemias of cats, cattle and some other mammals. Some forms of leukaemia in man are so like those of other species that a viral cause seems, by analogy, highly probable. It is not surprising that several workers have sought for, and found, virus-like particles in the blood of human leukaemias. Some of these have been said to resemble the C particles of murine leukaemias [281], others are probably the same as the EB virus of Burkitt's lymphoma and yet others are different again. The difficulty lies, not in accepting that the objects seen are viruses but in knowing whether they are likely to be causative agents or merely passengers, present by accident. We must admit that this approach to the problem has little value unless there is support from the use of other techniques.

Even if we cannot infect human beings with possible tumour viruses, one can try to infect human tissues in culture and look for transformation and other changes. As mentioned earlier, the SV 40 virus will transform human cells, though it has never been shown to cause human cancers. As yet, however, no success has been attained in revealing human cancer viruses by such techniques, very probably for the reason, mentioned above, that any virus present is not there in a free infectious state or is represented only by a remnant.

Immunological methods offer more hope. Even here, there are difficulties. Virus tumours in hamsters may be large enough to kill, yet no complement-fixing antibody may be detectable. Antibodies are more likely to be found in hosts with slow-growing tumours and in those with metastases. Accordingly, a group in the

USA has been collecting for subsequent careful study sera from selected patients with long-standing tumours [316]. These can be tested for antibody, as useful clues and opportunities arise. Of course many hosts with tumours of apparently non-virus origin do develop antibodies against extracts of their tumours and these are most commonly specific for the particular tumour, as discussed on p. 130. One cannot deduce that a virus is concerned in these; nor can one look for antibodies against wholly undiscovered viruses. It is more reasonable, if one suspects that a known virus might be involved, to look for evidence of possible T-antigens or transplantation antigens. For instance in Hong Kong, East Africa and other places in the tropics there is a high incidence of naso-pharyngal cancer. We know that adenoviruses normally inhabit the nasopharynx and that some adenovirus types are oncogenic. It is very reasonable, therefore, to look into the possibility that adenoviruses might, for some unknown reason, be particularly likely to produce cancers of the nasopharynx in the tropics. Among the adenoviruses, placed in three groups according to their antigen potency, just three T-antigens have been revealed. So it was not difficult to test for antibodies to these in the human sera. As it happens, all such tests so far have been negative. Nevertheless, we see here an example of an intelligent approach to the subject. When a virus is suspected but is not known to be oncogenic in animals, we have no readily available T-antigen against which to test our sera. Sabin and Todaro [316], using the herpes virus as an example, have shown how this difficulty might be overcome. We know that an antigen apparently identical with T-antigen is transiently present in virus infections which have no oncogenic outcome. So guinea pigs were injected with tissue cultures con-taining much herpes virus: the cultures had been harvested only three hours after infection at a time when 'early antigen' might be presumed to be present. Sera were obtained from these guinea pigs, then absorbed with sedimented virus obtained from late har-vests: they were found to contain an antibody reacting only with antigen from early harvests. Such a serum would be of use to test for a possible T-antigen in tumours suspected to be possibly due to herpes viruses.

One could go on asking more and more questions. Is there a

common biochemical lesion produced in cells both by viruses and by chemical or physical agents? Could such a finding lead to a unifying hypothesis bringing together all carcinogenic agents?

Final comments

We cannot conclude that cancers in general have a viral cause: the evidence is not there. Equally, we cannot conclude that the hypothesis is wrong: difficulties in the way of substantiating it are great and the facts are not in conflict with it. New techniques are being invented or perfected and may be capable of testing in new ways the correctness of the 'virus theory'. The evidence coming from the study of virus tumours in animals has been a major factor in causing a big change in thought about cancer. It is now a generally accepted view that the immunology of cancer is all-important, that cancer develops through failure of the mechanisms, largely immunological, which hold rebellious cells in check. Here lies great hope for the future. We can hope by immunological means to supplement and reinforce the efforts of surgeons and radiologists, so that their efforts are permanently successful and less frequently only temporary palliatives. We may hope to learn how to stimulate cellular defence mechanisms so that cancers have no chance to develop [234]. We know that histology can reveal in the prostate gland and elsewhere 'carcinoma *in situ*' – growths which look like cancer but remain under control and never spread. It has been reported that one can non-specifically stimulate immunity in mice with the attenuated tubercle bacillus BCG, so that tumour incidence is decreased [368]. One has now every reason to hope for more knowledge and practical benefits from studies of the immunology of cancer.

A final point must be made clear. If it turns out that viruses are concerned in causing many human cancers, it does not follow that it should be thought of and treated as an infectious disease. No credit is nowadays given to the old notion that there are 'cancer houses' in which successive inhabitants are likely to die of the disease. Human cancer viruses if they do exist, are likely to be widely occurring agents: their ability to lead to cancer probably depends on a variety of factors, not merely the presence of the virus. The occurrence of 'clusters' of cases of leukaemia in children (see p. 61) might have explanations other than those involving transmission of an infectious virus.

The intensive work now proceeding in many countries on the various lines described in this book allows us to hope that we shall soon know the answer to our as yet 'unanswered questions'.

References

1 ABERCROMBIE, M., & HEAYSMAN, J. E. M. (1954) Observations on the social behaviour of cells in tissue culture. 2. *Exp. cell res. 6:* 293

2 AHLSTRÖM, C. G., & ANDREWES, C. H. (1938) Fibroma virus infection in tarred rabbits. *J. Path. Bact. 47:* 65

3 ——, BERGMAN, S., & EHRENBERG, B. (1963) Neoplasms in guinea pigs induced by an agent in Rous chicken sarcoma. *Acta path. microbiol. scand. 58:* 177

4 ——, BERGMAN, S., FORSBY, N., & JONSSON, N. (1963) Rous sarcoma in mammals. *Acta un. int. Cancr. 19:* 294

5 —— & FORSBY, N. (1962) Sarcomas in hamsters after injection with Rous chicken tumor material. *J. exp. Med. 115:* 839

6 —— & JONSSON, N. (1962) Induction of sarcoma in rats by a variant of Rous virus. *Acta path. microbiol. scand. 54:* 145

7 ——, KATO, R., & LEVAN, A. (1964) Rous sarcoma in Chinese hamsters. *Science 144:* 1232

8 ALLISON, A. C. (1967) Cell-mediated immune responses to virus infections and virus-induced tumours. *Brit. med Bull. 23:* 60

9 —— (1968) I wish I knew. Do viruses cause cancer in man? *Lancet 1:* 1141

10 —— & FRIEDMAN, R. M. (1966) Effects of immune suppressants on Shope rabbit fibroma. *J. nat. Canc. Inst. 36:* 859

11 —— & LAW, L. (1968) Effects of antilymphocytic serum on virus oncogenesis. *Proc. Soc. exp. Biol.* (New York) *127:* 207

12 —— (1969) Immune responses to virus-induced tumours. *Proc. roy. Soc. Med. 62:* 956

13 ANDERVONT, H. B. (1952) Biological studies of the mammary-tumor inciter in mice. *Ann. N.Y. acad. Sci. 54:* 1004

14 ANNOTATION (1969) Immunosuppression and cancer. *Lancet 1:* 505

15 ANDREWES, C. H. (1931) The immunological relationships of fowl tumours with different histological structure. *J. Path. Bact. 34:* 91

16 —— (1932) The transmission of fowl tumours to pheasants. *Ibid. 35:* 407

17 —— (1933) The active immunization of pheasants against fowl tumours. *Ibid. 37:* 17.

18 —— (1933) Further serological studies on fowl tumour viruses. *Ibid. 37:* 27

19 —— (1934) Viruses in relation to the etiology of tumours. *Lancet 2:* 63 and 117

20 —— (1936) A change in rabbit fibroma suggesting mutation. 1. Experiments on domestic rabbits. *J. exp. Med. 63:* 157

21 —— (1936) Evidence for the presence of virus in a non-filterable tar sarcoma of the fowl. *J. Path. Bact. 63:* 23

22 —— (1939) The occurrence of neutralizing antibodies for Rous virus in the sera of young 'normal' chicks. *Ibid. 48:* 225

23 —— & AHLSTRÖM, C. G. (1938) A transplantable sarcoma occurring in a rabbit inoculated with tar and infectious fibroma virus. *Ibid. 47:* 87

24 ——, ——, FOULDS, L., & GYE, W. E. (1937) Reaction of tarred rabbits to the infectious fibroma virus (Shope). *Lancet 2:* 895

25 ——, ALLISON, A. C., ARMSTRONG, J. A., BEARCROFT, G., NIVEN, J. S. F., & PEREIRA, H. G. (1959) A virus disease of monkeys causing large superficial growths. *Acta un. int. Cancr. 15:* 760

26 —— & PEREIRA, H. G. (1967) *Viruses of vertebrates* (2nd ed.). Baillière, Tindall and Cassell

27 —— & SHOPE, R. E. (1936) A change in rabbit fibroma suggesting mutation. 3. Interpretation of findings. *J. exp. Med. 63:* 179

28 ATCHISON, R. W., CASTO, B. C., & HAMMON, W. McD. (1966) Electron microscopy of adeno-associated virus (AAV) in cell cultures. *Virology 29:* 353

29 BALLS, M. (1965) Lymphosarcoma in the South African clawed toad *Xenopus laevis*: a virus tumor. *Ann. N.Y. Acad. Sci. 126:* 256

30 —— & RUBEN, L. N. (1965) The transmission of lymphosarcoma in *Xenopus laevis*, the South African clawed toad. *Cancer Res. 27:* 654

31 BARSKI, G., & CORNEFORT-JENSEN, FR. (1966) Cytogenetic study of Sticker venereal sarcoma in European dogs. *J. nat. Canc. Inst. 37:* 787

32 BASSIN, R. H., SIMONS, P. J., CHESTERMAN, F. C., & HARVEY, J. J. (1968) Murine sarcoma virus (Harvey): characteristics of focus formation. *Int. J. Cancer 3:* 265

33 BEARCROFT, W. G. C., & JAMIESON, M. F. (1958) An outbreak of subcutaneous tumours in rhesus monkeys. *Nature* (London) *182:* 195

34 BEARD, J. W. (1956) The fallacy of the concept of virus masking. *Cancer Res. 16:* 279

35 —— & ROUS, P. (1934) A virus-induced mammalian growth with the characters of a tumour. 2. *J. exp. Med. 60:* 723

36 BELL, T. M. (1967) Viruses associated with Burkitt's tumour. *Progr. med Virol. 9:* 1

37 BERNHARD, W. (1958) Electron microscopy of tumor cells and tumor viruses. *Cancer Res. 18:* 491

38 BIGGS, P. M., & PAYNE, L. N. (1967) Studies on Marek's disease. 1. Experimental transmission. *J. nat. Canc. Inst. 39:* 267

39 BITTNER, J. J. (1936) Some possible effects of nursing on the mammary-gland tumour incidence in mice. *Science 84:* 162

40 BLACK, P. H. (1968) The oncogenic DNA viruses: a review of *in vitro* transformation studies. *Ann. Rev. Microbiol. 22:* 391

41 —— (1966) Transformation of mouse cell-line ... by SV 40. *Virology 28:* 760

42 —— & ROWE, W. P. (1963) An analysis of SV 40-induced transformation of hamster kidney tissue *in vitro*. 1. *Proc. nat. Acad. Sci.* (Washington) *50:* 606

43 BLAIR, P. B. (1968) The mammary-tumor virus (MTV). *Current topics in Microbiology 45:* 1. Springer-Verlag, Berlin

44 BOIRON, M., LÉVY, J. P., & PÉRIÈS, J. (1967) *In vitro* investigations on murine leukaemia viruses. *Progr. med. Virol. 9:* 341. S. Kargen, Basel and New York

45 ——, ——, THOMAS, M., FRIEDMAN, J. C., & BERNARD, J. (1964) Some properties of bovine papilloma virus. *Nature* (London) *201:* 423

46 BONAR, R. A., HEINE, V., BEARD, D., & BEARD, J. W. (1963) Virus of avian myeloblastosis (BAI strain A). 23. Morphology. *J. nat. Canc. Inst. 30:* 949

47 ——, PARSONS, D. F., BEAUDREAU, C. S., BECKER, C., & BEARD, J. W. (1959) Ultrastructure of avian myeloblasts in tissue culture. *J. nat. Canc. Inst. 23:* 199

48 BORREL, A. (1903) Epithélioses infectieuses et epithélioma. *Ann. Inst. Pasteur 17:* 81

49 BUBENIK, J., & BAUER, H. (1967) Antigenic characteristics of the interaction between Rous sarcoma virus and mammalian cells: complement-fixing and transplantation antigens. *Virology 31:* 489

50 BURKITT, D. (1958) A sarcoma involving the jaws of African children. *Brit. J. Surg. 46:* 218

51 BURMESTER, B. R., GROSS, M. A., WALTER, W. G., & FORTES, A. K. (1959) Pathogenicity of a viral strain (RPL 12) causing avian visceral lymphomatosis, and related neoplasms. 3. *J. nat. Canc. Inst. 22:* 107

52 BURNET, F. M. (1964) Immunological factors in carcinogenesis. *Brit. med. Bull. 20:* 154

53 CAME, P. E., & LUNGER, P. D. (1966) Viruses isolated from frogs and their relationship to the Lucké tumour. *Arch. ges. Virusforsch. 19:* 464

54 CARR, J. G. (1959) A survey of fowl tumours for induction of kidney carcinomas. *Virology 8:* 269

55 —— (1960) Lack of pathogenicity of Rous 1 virus for humans: a long-term experiment. *Vet. Record 72:* 87

56 CASALS, J. (1957) The arthropod-borne group of animal viruses. *Trans. N.Y. Acad. Sci. ser. 2 19:* 219

57 CHAMORRO, A., LATARJET, R., VIGIER, P., & ZAJDALA, F. (1962) New investigations on the Friend disease. In *Tumour viruses of murine origin* (CIBA symposium), p. 176. Churchill, London

58 CHANOCK, R. M., LUDWIG, W., HUEBNER, R. J., CATE, J. R., & CHU, L.-W. (1966) Immunization by selective infection with type 4 adenovirus grown in human diploid cells. *J. Amer. Med. Ass. 195:* 445

59 CHAPMAN, A. L., BOPP, W. I., BRIGHTWELL, A. S., COHEN, H., & NIELSEN, A. H. (1967) Preliminary report on virus-like particles in canine leukemia. *Cancer Res. 27:* 18

60 ——, BOPP, W., BRIGHTWELL, S., NIELSON & WERDER, A. (1966) Distribution of virus-like particles in the lymphatic tissues of non-leukemic CPWw conventional mice. *Proc. Soc. exp. Biol.* (New York) *123:* 742

61 CHRISTENSEN, L. R., BOND, E., & MATANIC, B. (1967) 'Pockless' rabbit pox. *Lab. Anim. Care 17:* 281

62 CHURCHILL, A. E., & BIGGS, P. M. (1967) Agent of Marek's disease in tissue culture. *Nature* (London) *215:* 528

63 ——, PAYNE, L. N., & CHUBB, R. C. (1969) Immunization against Marek's disease using a live attenuated virus. *Nature* (London) *221:* 744

64 CLAUDE, A. & MURPHY, J. B. (1933) Transmissible tumours of the fowl. *Physiol. Rev. 13:* 246

65 CLEMMESEN, J. (1929) The influence of Roentgen radiation on immunity to Shope fibroma virus. *Amer. J. Cancer 35:* 376

66 —— (1966) Epidemiological aspects of human leukemia. In *Comparative leukemia research*, p. 161. Pergamon Press, Oxford

67 COOK, R. H., & OLSON, C. (1951) Experimental transmission of cutaneous papilloma of the horse. *Amer. J. Path. 27:* 1087

68 COOPER, H. L., MACKAY, C. M., & BANFIELD, W. G. (1964) Chromosome studies of a contagious reticular-cell sarcoma of the Syrian hamster. *J. nat. Canc. Inst. 33:* 691

69 COWDRY, E. V. (1934) The problem of intranuclear inclusions in virus diseases. *Arch. Path. 18:* 527

70 DALLDORF, G., LINSELL, C. A., BARNHART, F. E., & MARTYN, R. (1964) An epidemiologic approach to the lymphomas of African children and Burkitt's sarcoma of the jaws. *Perspect. Biol. Med. 7:* 435

71 —— & SICKLES, G. M. (1948) An unidentified filterable agent isolated from the faeces of children with paralysis. *Science 108:* 61

72 DARLINGTON, R. W., GRANOFF, P. E., & BREEZE, D. C. (1966) Viruses and renal cancer of *Rana pipiens*: ultrastructural studies. *Virology 29:* 149

73 DAWSON, P. J., TACKE, R. B., & FIELDSTEEL, A. H. (1968) Relationship between Friend virus and an associated lymphatic leukaemia virus. *Brit. J. Canc. 22:* 569

74 DEFENDI, V., & LEHMAN, J. M. (1964) The nature of the haemorrhagic lesions induced by polyoma virus in hamsters. *Cancer Res. 24:* 329

75 ——, EPHRUSSI, B., KOPROWSKI, H., & YOSHIDA, M. C. (1965) Properties of hybrids between polyoma-transformed and normal mouse cells. *Proc. nat. Acad. Sci.* (Washington) *57:* 299

76 DE HARVEN, E., & FRIEND, C. (1964) Study of virus particles partially purified from the blood of leukemic mice. *Virology 23:* 119

77 DEICHMAN, G. I., & KLUCHAREVA, T. E. (1966) Loss of transplantation antigen in primary simian-virus-40-induced tumors and their metastases. *J. nat. Canc. Inst. 36:* 647

78 DEINHARDT, F. (1966) Neoplasms induced by Rous sarcoma virus in new-world monkeys. *Nature* (London) *210:* 443

79 DE MAEYER, E., & DE MAEYER-GUIGNARD, J. (1968) Effect of different carcinogenic agents on the production of interferon in tissue culture and in the animal. In *Interferon* (CIBA foundation symposium), p. 218. Churchill, London

80 DENT, P. B., COOPER, M. D., PAYNE, L. N., GOOD, R. A., & BURMESTER, B. R. (1967) Characterization of avian lymphoid leukosis as a malignancy of the bursal lymphoid system. *Perspectives in Virology: 5:* 257. Academic Press, New York and London

81 DES LIGNERIS, M. J. A. (1931) On the transplantation of Rous fowl sarcoma No. 1 into guinea-fowls and turkeys. *Amer. J. Cancer 16:* 307

82 DIDERHOLM, H., BERG, R., & WESSLÉN, T. (1966) Transformation of rat and guinea pig cells *in vitro* by SV 40. *Int. J. Cancer 1:* 139

83 DOUGHERTY, R. M., & DI STEFANO, H. W. (1966) Lack of relationship between infection with avian leukosis virus and the presence of COFAL antigen in chick embryos. *Virology 29:* 586

84 DOURMASHKIN, R. R., & SIMONS, P. J. (1961) The ultrastructure of Rous sarcoma virus. *J. Ultrastruct. Res. 5:* 505

85 DUBREUIL, R., DI FRANCO, E., PAVILANIS, V., & MAROIS, P. (1967) Tumeurs à virus SV 40. *Canad. J. Microbiol. 13:* 1433

86 DUFF, R. G., & VOGT, P. K. (1969) Characteristics of two new avian tumor virus subgroups. *Virology 39:* 18

87 DULBECCO, R. & VOGT, M. (1960) Significance of continual virus production in tissue cultures rendered neoplastic by polyoma virus. *Proc. nat. Acad. Sci.* (Washington) *46:* 1617

88 DUNGERN, E. VON & COCA, A. F. (1903) Hare sarcomas growing in rabbits and the nature of tumor immunity. *Z. ImmunForsch. 2:* 391

89 DURAN-REYNALS, F. (1940) A haemorrhagic disease occurring in chickens inoculated with the Rous and Fujinami viruses. *Yale J. Biol. Med. 13:* 77

90 —— (1942) The reciprocal infection of ducks and chickens with tumor-inducing viruses. *Cancer Res. 2:* 343

91 —— (1943) The infection of turkeys and guinea-fowl by the Rous sarcoma virus and the accompanying variations of the virus. *Ibid. 3:* 569

92 —— (1945) Immunological factors that influence the neoplastic effects of the rabbit fibroma. *Ibid. 5:* 25

93 —— (1957) Studies on the combined effects of chemical carcinogens, hormones and virus infections. *Texas Rep. on Biol. and Med. 15:* 306

94 —— & BRYAN, E. (1952) Studies on combined effects of fowl-pox virus and methylcholanthrene in chickens. *Ann. N.Y. Acad. Sci. 54:* 977

95 DUTCHER, R. M., LARKIN, E. P., TUMILOWICZ, J. J., MARSHAK, R. R., & SZEKELY, I. E. (1966) Recent studies in bovine leukemia. *Comparative leukemia research,* p. 37. Pergamon Press, Oxford

96 ——, SZEKELY, I. E., BARTIE, B. W., & SWITZER, J. W. (1964) Attempts to demonstrate a virus for bovine lymphosarcoma. *Amer. J. Vet. Res. 25:* 668

97 ECKERT, E. A., ROTH, R., & SCHÄFER, W. (1963) Myxovirus-like structure of avian myeloblastosis virus. *Z. Naturforsch. 18B:* 339

98 EDDY, B., BORMAN, G. S., GRUBBS, G. E., & YOUNG, R. D. (1961) Identification of the oncogenic substance in rhesus monkey kidney as simian virus 40. *Virology 17:* 65

99 ——, ROWE, W. P., HARTLEY, J. W., STEWART, S. E., & HUEBNER, R. T. (1958) Haemagglutination with the SE polyoma virus. *Virology 6:* 290

100 ——, STEWART, S. E., KIRSCHSTEIN, R. L., & YOUNG, R. D. (1959) Induction of subcutaneous nodules in rabbits with the SE polyoma virus. *Nature* (London) *183:* 766

101 ELFORD, W. J., & ANDREWES, C. H. (1935) Estimation of the size of a fowl tumour virus by filtration through graded membranes. *Brit. J. exp. Path. 16:* 61

102 ELLERMAN, V., & BANG, O. (1908) Experimentelle Leukämie bei Hühnern. *Centralbl. Bakt. 46:* 595

103 ENDERS, J. F., & DIAMANDOPOULOS G. TH. (1969) A study of variation and progression in oncogenicity in an SV 40-transformed hamster-heart cell-line and its clones. *Proc. Roy. Soc.* (B) *171:* 431

104 EPSTEIN, M. A., & ACHONG, B. G. (1965) Specific immunofluorescence test for herpes-type EB virus of Burkitt lymphoblasts. *J. nat. Canc. Inst. 40:* 593

105 ——, ——, & BARR, Y. M. (1964) Virus particles in cultured lymphoblasts from Burkitt's lymphoma. *Lancet 1:* 702

106 ——, HENLE, G., ACHONG, B. G., & BARR, Y. M. (1965) Morphological and biological studies on a virus in cultured lymphoblasts from Burkitt's lymphoma. *J. exp. Med. 121:* 761

107 ——, WOODALL, J. P., & THOMSON, A. D. (1964) Lymphoblastic lymphoma in the bone marrow of African green monkeys (*C. aethiops*) inoculated with biopsy material from a child with Burkitt's lymphoma. *Lancet 2:* 288

108 EPSTEIN, W. L., FUKUYAMO, K., & BENN, M. (1968) Transmission of a pigmented melanoma in golden hamsters by a cell-free ultrafiltrate. *Nature* (London) *219:* 979

109 FEFER, A., McCOY, J. L., & GLYNN, J. P. (1967) Induction and regression of primary mouse-sarcoma-virus-induced tumors in mice. *Cancer Res. 27:* 1626

110 FELLUGA, B., CLAUDE, A., & MRENA, E. (1969) Electron-microscopic observations on virus particles associated with a transplantable renal adenocarcinoma. *J. nat. Canc. Inst. 43:* 319

111 FENNER, F. (1968) *The biology of animal viruses,* p. 26. Academic Press, New York and London

112 —— *Ibid.,* p. 649

113 —— *Ibid.,* p. 667

114 FIELDSTEEL, A. H., KURAHARA, C., & DAWSON, P. J. (1969) Moloney leukaemia virus as a helper in retrieving Friend virus from a non-infectious reticular sarcoma. *Nature* (London) *223:* 1274

115 FINCH, J. T., & KLUG, A. (1965) The structure of viruses of the papilloma–polyoma group. 3. Structure of rabbit papilloma virus. *J. molec. Biol. 13:* 1

116 FINKEL, M. P., BISKIS, B. O., & JINKINS, P. B. (1966) Viral induction of osteosarcomas in mice. *Science 151:* 698

117 ——, ——, & FARRELL, C. (1968) Osteosarcomas appearing in hamsters after treatment with extracts of human osteosarcomas. *Proc. nat. Acad. Sci.* (Washington) *60:* 1223

118 FISCHINGER, P. J., & O'CONNOR, T. E. (1969) Isolation and identification of a helper virus found in the Moloney-sarcoma–leukemia complex. *Science 165:* 714

119 FOULDS, L. (1954) The experimental study of tumor progression. *Cancer Res. 14:* 327

120 FRIEDEWALD, W. F., & ROUS, P. (1944) The initiating and promoting elements in tumour production. *J. exp. Med. 80:* 101

121 FRIEND, C. (1957) Cell-free transmission in adult mice of a disease having the character of a leukemia. *J. exp. Med. 105:* 307

122 FUJINAMI, A., & HATANO, S. (1929) Contribution of the pathology of tumor: a duck sarcoma from chicken sarcoma. *Gann. 23:* 67

123 FURMINGER, K. G. S., & BEALE, A. J. (1968) The complement-fixation test for avian leukosis. *J. gen. Virol. 3:* 25

124 FURTH, J. (1931) Erythroleukosis and the anaemias of the fowl. *Arch. Path. 12:* 1

125 —— (1933) Lymphoblastosis, myelomatosis and endothelioma of chickens caused by a filterable agent. 1. *J. exp. Med. 58:* 253

126 GALIBERT, F., BERNARD, C., CHENAILLE, P. H., & BOIRON, M. (1966) Investigation of Rauscher-virus nucleic acid. *Nature* (London) *209:* 680

127 GAUGAS, J. M., CHESTERMAN, F. C., HIRSCH, M. S., REES, R. J. W., HARVEY, J. J., & GILCHRIST, C. (1969) Unexpected high incidence of tumors in thymectomized mice treated with antilymphocytic serum and *Mycobacterium leprae*. *Nature* (London) *221:* 1033

128 GEERING, G., HARDY, W. D., OLD, L. J., DE HARVEN, E., & BRODEY, R. S. (1968) Shared group-specific antigen of murine and feline leukemia viruses. *Virology 36:* 678

129 GERALDES, A. (1969) Malignant transformation of hamster cells by cell-free extracts of bovine papillomas *in vitro*. *Nature* (London) *222:* 1283

130 GERBER, P. (1964) Virogenic hamster tumor cells: induction of virus synthesis. *Science 145:* 833

131 —— & BIRCH, S. M. (1967) Complement-fixing antibodies in sera . . . to virus antigens derived from Burkitt's lymphoma cells. *Proc. nat. Acad. Sci.* (Washington) *58:* 478

132 —— & KIRSCHSTEIN, R. L. (1962) SW 40-induced ependymomas in newborn hamsters. 1. *Virology 18:* 582

133 GINSBERG, H. S., PEREIRA, H. G., VALENTINE, R. C., & WILCOX, W. C. (1966) A proposed terminology for the adenovirus antigens and virion morphological units. *Virology 28:* 782

134 GIRARDI, A. J., & JENSEN, F. C. (1966) Transformation of human cells by oncogenic virus SV 40. In *Malignant transformation by viruses*, p. 124. Springer-Verlag, Berlin

135 GOODPASTURE, E. W., & TEAGUE, O. (1923) Experimental production of herpetic lesions in organs and tissues of the rabbit. *J. med. Res. 44:* 121

136 GORDON, D. E., & OLSON, C. (1968) Meningiomas and fibroblastic neoplasia in calves induced with the bovine papilloma virus. *Cancer Res. 28:* 2423

137 GRACE, J. T., MIRAND, E. A., MILLIAN, S. J., & METZGER, R. S. (1962) Experimental studies of human tumors. *Fed. Proc. 21:* 32

138 GRAFFI, A. (1957) Chloroleukemia of mice. *Ann. N.Y. Acad. Sci. 68:* 540

139 ——, SCHRAMM, T., BENDER, E., et al. (1967) Ueber einen neuen

virushaltigen Hauttumor beim Goldhamster. *Arch. Geschwulstforsch* 30: 277

140 ——, ——, ——, GRAFFI, I., HORN, K. H., & BIERWOLF, D. (1968). Cell-free transmissible leukoses in Syrian hamsters, probably of viral etiology. *Brit. J. Cancer* 22: 577

141 ——, ——, GRAFFI, I., BIERWOLF, D., & BENDER, E. (1968) Virus-associated skin tumours of the Syrian hamster. *J. nat. Canc. Inst.* 40: 867

142 GRANOFF, A., CAME, P. E., & BREEZE, D. C. (1966) Viruses and renal carcinoma of *Rana pipiens*. 1. The isolation and properties of viruses from normal and tumor tissue. *Virology* 29: 133

143 GREEN, M., & PIÑA, M. (1964) Biochemical studies on adenovirus multiplication. 6. Properties of highly purified tumorigenic human adenoviruses and their DNAs. *Proc. nat. Acad. Sci.* (Washington) 51: 1251

144 GRESSER, I., & seven others. The effect of interferon preparations on Friend leukaemia in mice. In *Interferon* (CIBA foundation symposium), p. 240. Churchill, London

145 GROSS, L. (1951) 'Spontaneous' leukaemia developing in C3H mice following inoculation in infancy with AK leukemic extracts or AK embyros. *Proc. Soc. exp. Biol.* (New York) 76: 27

146 —— (1957) Influence of ether, *in vitro*, on pathogenic properties of mouse leukemic extracts. *Acta haemat.* 15: 273

147 —— (1962) Studies on pathogenic properties and natural transmission of a mouse leukemia virus. In *Tumour viruses of murine origin* (CIBA foundation symposium), p. 159. Churchill, London

148 —— (1966) The Rauscher virus: a mixture of the Friend virus and of the mouse leukemia virus (Gross). *Acta haemat.* 35: 200

149 GUSEV, A. T., & SVOBODA, J. (1962) Comparison of Rous sarcoma with sarcoma XC by precipitation in agar. *Folia biol.* (Prague) 8: 140

150 GYE, W. E. (1931) A note on the propagation of Fujinami's fowl myxosarcoma in ducks. *Brit. J. exp. Path.* 12: 93

151 —— (1932) The propagation of Fujinami's fowl myxosarcoma in ducklings. *Ibid.* 13: 458

152 —— & ANDREWES, C. H. (1924) A study of the Rous sarcoma No. 1. 1. Filterability. *Ibid.* 7: 81

153 —— & BARNARD, J. E. (1925) New research into the origin of cancer. *Lancet* 2: 81

154 —— & PURDY, W. J. (1931) *The cause of cancer*. Cassell, London

155 HABEL, K. (1961) Resistance of polyoma-immune animals to transplanted polyoma tumours. *Proc. Soc. exp. Biol.* (New York) 106: 722

156 HADDOW, A. J. (1963) An improved map for the study of Burkitt's lymphoma in Africa. *E. Afr. med. J.* 40: 429

157 —— (1964) Age incidence in Burkitt's lymphoma syndrome. *Ibid.* 41: 1

158 HANAFUSA, H., HANAFUSA, T., & RUBIN, H. (1963) The defectiveness of Rous sarcoma virus. *Proc. nat. Acad. Sci* (Washington) 49: 572

159 HAREL, J. (1956) Role de la résistance naturelle dans l'evolution des

tumours provoquées par le virus fibromateux de Shope. *C.r. Soc. Biol.* (Paris) *150:* 357

160 HARRIS, H. MILLER, O. J., KLEIN, G., WORST, P., & TACHIBANA, T. (1969) Suppression of malignancy by cell fusion. *Nature* (London) *223:* 363

161 HARRIS, R. J. C., CHESTERMAN, F. C., & NEGRONI, G. (1961) Induction of tumours in newborn ferrets with Mill Hill polyoma virus. *Lancet 1:* 788

162 —— & SIMONS, P. J. (1958) Nature of the antigens responsible for the acquired tolerance of turkeys to Rous sarcoma agent. *Nature* (London) *181:* 1485

163 HARTLEY, J. W., & ROWE, W. P. (1964) New papovavirus contaminating Shope papilloma. *Science 143:* 258

164 —— & —— (1966) Production of altered cell foci in tissue culture by defective Moloney sarcoma virus particles. *Proc. nat. Acad. Sci.* (Washington) *55:* 780

165 ——, ——, CAPPS, W. L., & HUEBNER, R. J. (1969) Isolation of naturally occurring viruses of the murine leukemic group in tissue culture. *J. Virol. 3:* 126

166 HARVEY, J. J. (1965) An unidentified virus which causes the rapid production of tumours in mice. *Nature* (London) *204:* 1104

167 HELLSTRÖM, I., HELLSTRÖM, K. C., EVANS, C. A., HEPPNER, G.H., PIERCE, G. E., & YANG, J. P. S. (1969) Serum-mediated protection of neoplastic cells from inhibition by lymphocytes immune to their tumor-specific antigens. *Proc. nat. Acad. Sci.* (Washington) *62:* 362

168 HENLE, G., HENLE, W., & DIEHL, V. (1968) Relation of Burkitt's tumor-associated herpes-type virus to infectious mononucleosis. *Proc. nat. Acad. Sci.* (Washington) *59:* 94

169 HENLE, W., DIEHL, V., KOHN, G., ZUR HAUSEN, H., & HENLE, G. (1967) Herpes-type virus chromosome marker in normal leukocytes after growth with irradiated Burkitt cells. *Science 157:* 1064

170 HEPPNER, G. H. (1967) The effect of thymectomy on the development of nodules and tumours induced by the mouse tumor virus. *Proc. Am. Ass. Cancer Res. 8:* 27

171 HILLEMAN, M. R. (1966) Approaches to control of cancer by immunological procedures. In *Comparative leukemia research,* p. 105. Pergamon Press, Oxford

172 HOLOWCZAK, J. A., & JOKLIK, W. K. (1967) Studies on the structural proteins of vaccinia virus. 2. *Virology 33:* 726

173 HUEBNER, R. J. (1967) Adenovirus-directed tumor and T-antigens. *Perspectives in Virology 5:* 147. Academic Press, New York and London

174 ——, CHANOCK, R. M., RUBIN, B. A., & CASEY, M. J. (1964) Induction by adenovirus 7 of tumors in hamsters having the antigenic characters of SV 40 virus. *Proc. nat. Acad. Sci.* (Washington) *52:* 1333

175 ——, PEREIRA, H. G., ALLISON, A. C., HOLLINSHEAD, A. C., & TURNER, H. E. (1964) Production of type-specific C antigen in virus-free hamster tumor cells induced by adenovirus type 12. *Proc. nat. Acad. Sci.* (Washington) *51:* 432

176 ——, HARTLEY, J. W., ROWE, W. P., LANE, W. T., & CAPPS, W. I. (1966) Rescue of the defective genome of Moloney sarcoma virus from a non-infectious hamster tumour. *Proc. nat. Acad. Sci.* (Washington) *56:* 1164

177 ——, ROWE, W. P., HARTLEY, J. W., & LANE, W. T. (1962) Mouse polyoma virus in a rural ecology. In *Tumour viruses of murine origin* (CIBA foundation symposium), p. 314. Churchill, London

178 ——, ——, & LANE, W. T. (1962) Oncogenic effects in hamsters of adenoviruses types 12 and 18. *Proc. nat. Acad. Sci.* (Washington) *48:* 2051

179 JARRETT, O. (1966) Different transplantation antigens in BHK 21 cells transformed by four strains of polyoma virus. *Virology 30:* 744

180 JARRETT, W. F. H., CRAWFORD, E. M., MARTIN, W. B., & DAVIE, F. (1964) A virus-like particle associated with leukaemia (lymphosarcoma). *Nature* (London) *202:* 567

181 ——, MARTIN, W. B., CRIGHTON, G. W., DALTON, R. G., & STEWART, M. F. (1964) Leukaemia in the cat: transmission experiments with leukaemia (lymphosarcoma). *Ibid. 202:* 566

182 JOHNSON, M., & MORA, P. T. (1967) Lipids of the Rauscher mouse leukemia virus. *Virology 31:* 230

183 JONSSON, N., & SJÖGREN, H. E. (1965) Further studies on specific transplantation antigens in Rous sarcoma of mice. *J. exp. Med. 122:* 403

184 —— (1956) Isograft resistance to Rous sarcomas in mice inoculated with Rous chicken sarcoma when newborn. *Exp. cell. res. 40:* 159

185 KAKUK, T. J., HINZ, R. W., LANGHAM, R. F., & CONNER, G. H. (1968) Experimental transmission of canine malignant lymphoma to the beagle neonate. *Cancer Res. 28:* 716

186 KAPLAN, H. S. (1967) On the natural history of the murine leukemias. *Cancer Res. 27:* 1325

187 KATO, S., ONO, K., MIYAMOTO, H., & MANTANI, M. (1966) Virus-host-cell interaction in rabbit fibrosarcoma produced by Shope fibroma. *Biken J. 9:* 57

188 KELLOFF, G. J., LANE, W. T., TURNER, H. E., & HUEBNER, R. J. (1969) *In vivo* studies of the FBJ murine osteosarcoma virus. *Nature* (London) *223:* 1379

189 KEOGH, E. V. (1938) Ectodermal lesions produced by the virus of Rous sarcoma. *Brit. J. exp. Path. 19:* 1

190 KIDD, J. (1938) Immunological reactions with a virus causing papillomas in rabbits. 1. Demonstration of a complement-fixation reaction. *J. exp. Med. 68:* 703

191 —— & ROUS, P. (1938) The carcinogenic effect of a papilloma virus on the tarred skin of rabbits. 2. *Ibid.* 529

192 KILHAM, L. (1955) Metastasizing viral fibroma of grey squirrels: pathogenesis and mosquito transmission. *Amer. J. Hyg. 61:* 55

193 —— & FISHER, E. R. (1954) Pathogenesis of fibromas in cottontail rabbits *Ibid. 59:* 104

194 ——, HERMAN, C. M., & FISHER, E. R. (1953) Naturally occurring fibromas of grey squirrels related to Shope's fibroma virus. *Proc. Soc. exp. Biol.* (New York) *82:* 298

195 KING, J. W., & DURAN-REYNALS, F. (1943) Development by ducks of natural neutralizing antibodies for a duck variant of the Rous sarcoma virus. *Yale J. Biol. Med. 16:* 53

196 KIRSCHSTEIN, R. I., RABSON, A. S., & KILHAM, L. (1958) Pulmonary lesions produced by fibroma viruses in squirrels and rabbits. *Cancer Res. 18:* 1340

197 KIRSTEN, W. H., MAYER, L. A., WOHLMANN, R. L., & PIERCE, M. I. (1967) Studies on a murine erythroblastosis virus. *J. nat. Canc. Inst. 38:* 117

198 KIT, S. (1967) In *Molecular biology of viruses*, p. 495. Academic Press, New York and London

199 KLEIN, G. (1966) Tumor antigens. *Ann. Rev. Microbiol. 20:* 223

200 ——, CLIFFORD, P., KLEIN, E., & STJERNSWARD, J. (1966) Search for tumor-specific immune reactions in Burkitt lymphoma patients by the membrane immunofluorescent method. *Proc. nat. Acad. sci.* (Washington) *55:* 1628

201 —— & KLEIN, E. (1964) Antigenic properties of lymphomas induced by the Moloney agent. In *Specific tumour antigens*, p. 82. Munkgaard: Copenhagen

202 KLEMENT, V., & SVOBODA, J. (1963) Successful induction of tumours in Syrian hamsters with cell-free Rous sarcoma filtrate. *Folia biol.* (Prague) *10:* 321

203 KLINKE, J. (1937) Die carcinogene Wirkung des 1,2-Benzpyrens am Kaninchen. *Z. Krebsforsch. 46:* 334

204 KLUG, A. (1968) Structure of viruses of the papilloma–polyoma type by tilting experiments: two-side images. *J. molec. Biol. 31:* 1

205 —— & FINCH, J. T. (1965) Structure of viruses of the papilloma-polyoma type 1. Human wart virus. *J. molec. Biol. 11:* 403

206 KOPROWSKI, H. (1966) The emperor's new clothes, or an inquiry into the present status of tumor viruses and virus tumors. In *Harvey lectures, series 60*, p. 173. Academic Press, New York

207 —— & NORTON, T. (1950) Interference between certain neurotropic viruses and transplantable mouse tumors. *Cancer* (Philadelphia) *3:* 874

208 ——,PONTEN, J. A., JENSEN, F., RAVDIN, R. G., MOORHEAD, P., & SAKSELA, E. (1962) Transformation of cultures of human tissue infected with simian virus SV 40. *J. cell. comp. Physiol. 59:* 281

209 KOSIROWSKA, J., & ZAKRZEWSKI, K. (1966) On the neoplastic transformation induced by vaccinia virus in primary cultures of mouse embryros. *Bull. Acad. pol. Sci. Sér. Sci. biol. 14:* 737

210 KREIDER, J. W., BREEDIS, C., & CURRAN, J. S. (1967) Interactions of Shope papilloma virus and rabbit skin cells *in vitro*. 1. *J. nat. Canc. Inst. 38:* 921

211 KRYUKOVA, I. N., OBUCH, I. B., & BIRYULINA, T. I. (1968) Tumour production in adult mice by syngeneic cultured cells containing the incomplete Rous virus. *Nature* (London) *219:* 174

212 LACASSAGNE, A. (1932) Apparition de cancers de la mamelle chez la souris male, soumise à des injections de folliculine. *C.r. Acad. Sci.* (Paris) *195:* 630

213 LANDON, J. G., ELLIS, L. B., ZEVA, V. H., & FAKIZIA, D. P. A.

(1968) Herpes-type virus in cultured leucocytes from chimpanzees. *J. nat. Canc. Inst. 40:* 181

214 LASFARGUES, E. Y., & MOORE, D. H. (1966) Cell transformation by the mammary-tumor virus *in vitro*. In *Malignant transformation by viruses*, p. 44. Springer-Verlag, Berlin

215 LAW, L. W. (1962) Influence of foster nursing on virus-induced and spontaneous leukemia in mice. *Proc. Soc. exp. Biol.* (New York) *111:* 615

216 —— (1965) Neoplasms in thymectomized mice following room infection with polyoma virus. *Nature* (London) *205:* 672

217 LEINATI, L., CILLI, V., MANDELLI, G., CASTRUCCI, G., CARRARA, O. & SCATOZZA, F. (1961) Anatomo-histopathological and virological researches on the nodular skin disease of the hares of the Po valley. *Bull. Ist. Sieroterap. Milan 40:* 295

218 LEVY, H. B., LAW, L. W., & RABSON, A. S. (1969) Inhibition of tumor growth by polyinosinic-polycytidylic acid. *Proc. nat. Acad. Sci.* (Washington) *62:* 357

219 LEVY, J. A., HENLE, G., HENLE, W., & ZAJAC, B. A. (1968) Effect of reovirus 3 on cultivated Burkitt tumour cells. *Nature* (London) *220:* 608

220 LIEBERMAN, M., and KAPLAN, H. S. (1959) Leukemogenic activity of filtrates from radiation-induced lymphoid tumors of mice. *Science 130:* 387

221 LUCKÉ, B. (1934) A neoplastic disease of the kidney of the frog, *Rana pipiens*. *Amer. J. Cancer 20:* 352

222 —— (1938) Carcinoma in the leopard frog: its probable causation by a virus. *J. exp. Med. 68:* 457

223 LYELL, A., & MILES, J. A. R. (1951) The myrmecia: a study of inclusion bodies in warts. *Brit. Med. J. 1:* 912

224 LYONS, M. J., & MOORE, D. H. (1965) Isolation of the mammary-tumor virus: chemical and morphological studies. *J. nat. Canc. Inst. 35:* 549

225 McINTOSH, J. (1933) On the nature of the tumours induced in fowls by injections of tar. *Brit. J. exp. Path. 14:* 422

226 MACKAY, J. M. K. (1969) Tissue-culture studies of sheep pulmonary adenomatosis (jaagsiekte). *J. comp. Path. 79:* 141 and 147

227 MACPHERSON, I. (1963) Characteristics of a hamster-cell clone transformed by polyoma virus. *J. nat. Canc. Inst. 30:* 795

228 —— (1966) In *Malignant transformation by viruses*, p. 1. Springer-Verlag, Berlin

229 —— & MONTAGNIER, L. (1964) Agar suspension culture for the selective assay of cells transformed by polyoma virus. *Virology 23:* 291

230 MAHY, W. I., HARVEY, J. J., & ROWSON, K. E. K. (1966) Some physical properties of a murine sarcoma virus (Harvey). *Texas Rep. Biol. Med. 24:* 620

231 MARIN, G., & MACPHERSON, I. (1969) Reversion in polyoma-transformed cells: retransformation, induced antigens and tumorigenicity. *J. Virol. 3:* 146

232 MARSHAK, R. R., ABT, D. A., & COHEN, D. (1966) Epidemiological

aspects of leukemia in animals. In *Comparative leukemia research*, p. 181. Pergamon Press, Oxford

233 MARSHALL, I. D., & REGNERY, D. R. (1960) Myxomatosis in a Californian brush rabbit (*Sylvilagus bachmani*). *Nature* (London) *188*: 73

234 MATHÉ, G., & seven others (1969) Active immunotherapy for acute lymphoblastic leukaemia. *Lancet 1*: 697

235 MELNICK, J. L. (1962) Papovavirus group. *Science 135*: 1128

236 —— & RAPP, F. (1965) Possible relationship between two primate papovaviruses, human wart and simian SV 40. *J. nat. Canc. Inst. 34*: 529

237 METCALF, D., FURTH, J., & BUFFETT, R. F. (1959) Pathogenesis of mouse leukemia caused by Friend virus. *Cancer Res. 19*: 52

238 MIDLIGE, F. H., & MALSBERGER, R. G. (1968) *In vitro* morphology and maturation of lymphocystis virus. *J. Virol. 2*: 830

239 MILLER J. F. A. P. (1962) Role of the thymus in virus-induced leukaemia. In *Tumour viruses of murine origin* (CIBA foundation symposium), p. 262. Churchill, London

240 MIRAND, E. A., & GRACE, J. T. (1962) Transmission of Friend disease from infected mothers to offspring. *Virology 16*: 344

241 ——, STEEVES, R. A., AVILA, L., & GRACE, J. T. (1968) Spleen focus formation by polycythaemic strains of Friend leukemia virus. *Proc. exp. Biol.* (New York) *127*: 900

242 MIZELL, M., STACKPOLE, C. W., & HALPEREN, S. (1968) Herpes-type virus recovery from 'virus-free' frog kidney tumors. *Proc. Soc. exp. Biol.* (New York) *127*: 808

243 MOLONEY, J. B. (1960) Biological studies on a lymphoid leukemia virus extracted from sarcoma 37. 1. Origin. *J. nat. Canc. Inst. 24*: 933

244 —— (1962) The rodent leukemias: virus-induced murine leukemias. *Fed. Proc. 21*: 9

245 —— (1966) A virus-induced rhabdomyosarcoma of mice. *Nat. Canc. Inst. monograph no. 22*, p. 139

246 MOMMAERTS, E. B., SHARP, D. G., ECKERT, E. A., BEARD, D., & BEARD, J. W. (1954) Virus of avian erythroblastic leukosis. *J. nat. Canc. Inst. 14*: 1011

247 MOORE, A. E. (1954) Effects of viruses on tumors. *Ann. Rev. Microbiol. 8*: 393

248 —— (1963) Consideration of means for determining if viruses are causally related to cancer in man. *Progr. med. Virol. 5*: 295

249 MOORE, D. H. (1962) On the identification and characterization of the milk agent. In *Tumour viruses of murine origin* (CIBA foundation symposium), p. 167. Churchill, London

250 —— & LYONS, M. J. (1964) The role of viruses in breast cancer causation. *Fifth Nat. Cancer Conf. Philadelphia*, p. 143. Lippincott

251 MORGAN, H. R. (1968) Antibodies for Rous sarcoma virus in fowl, animal and human populations in East Africa. *J. nat. Canc. Inst. 38*: 1229

252 MORTON, D. L., & MALMGREN, R. A. (1968) Human osteosarcomas: immunological evidence suggesting an associated infectious agent. *Science 162*: 1279

References 153

253 MUNROE, J. S., & WINDLE, W. F. (1963) Tumours induced in primates by chicken sarcoma viruses. *Science 140:* 1415

254 —— & —— (1966) Nephritis and brain atrophy in monkeys receiving chicken sarcoma viruses. Academic Press, New York and London

255 NAHMIAS, A. J. (1969) Association of genital herpes virus with cervical cancer. *Int. Virology 1:* 187

256 NAIB, Z. M., NAHMIAS, A. J., & JOSEY, W. R. (1966) Cytology and histopathology of cervical herpes simplex infection. *Cancer* (Philadelphia) *19:* 1026

257 NANDI, S. (1967) The histocompatibility-2 locus and susceptibility to Bittner virus borne by red blood cells in mice. *Proc. nat Acad. Sci.* (Washington) *58:* 485

258 NEGRONI, G. (1964) Isolation of viruses from leukaemic patients. *Brit. Med. J. 1:* 927

259 NIEDERMAN, J. C., McCOLLUM, R. W., HENLE, G., & HENLE, W. (1968) Infectious mononucleosis: clinical manifestations in relation to EB virus antibodies. *J. Amer. Med. Ass. 203:* 205

260 NIVEN, J. S. F., ARMSTRONG, J. A., ANDREWES, C. H., PEREIRA, H. G., & VALENTINE, R. C. (1961) Subcutaneous 'growths' in monkeys produced by a poxvirus. *J. Path. Bact. 81:* 1

261 NOBEL, T. A., NEUMANN, F., & KLOPFER, U. (1969) Histological patterns of metastases from pulmonary adenomatosis of sheep (jaagsiekte). *J. comp. Path. 79:* 537

262 NOYES, W. F. (1959) Studies in the Shope rabbit papilloma. 2. The location of infective virus in papillomas of the cottontail rabbit. *J. exp. Med. 109:* 423

263 O'CONNOR, T. E., & FISCHINGER, P. J. (1968) Titration patterns of a murine sarcoma–leukemia virus complex. *Science 159:* 325

264 —— & —— (1969) Physical properties of competent and defective states of a murine sarcoma (Moloney). *J. nat. Canc. Inst. 43:* 487

265 ODAKA, T., & IKAWA, Y. (1968) Friend-virus-induced transplantable tumours of C57 BL/6 origin containing small amounts of infectious virus. *Int. J. Canc. 3:* 211

266 OLD, L. J., & BOYSE, E. A. (1965) Antigens of tumours and leukemias produced by viruses. *Fed. Proc. 24:* 1009

267 ——, ——, OETTGEN, H. F., DE HARVEN, E., GEERING, G., WILLIAMSON, B., & CLIFFORD, P. Precipitating antibody in human serum to an antigen present in cultured Burkitt lymphoma cells. *Proc. nat. Acad. Sci.* (Washington) *56:* 1699

268 OLSON, C., & COOK, R. H. (1961) Cutaneous sarcoma-like lesions of the horse caused by the agent of bovine papilloma. *Proc. Soc. exp. Biol.* (New York) *77:* 281

269 ——, SEGAL, D., & SKIDMORE, L. V. (1960) Further observations on immunity to bovine cutaneous papillomatosis. *Amer. J. vet. Res. 21:* 233

270 OPLER, S. R. (1967) The pathology of cavian leukemia. *Amer. J. Path. 51:* 1135 and 1161

271 —— (1967) Animal model of viral oncogenesis. *Nature* (London) *215:* 184

272 OSATO, T., & ITO, Y. (1968) Immunofluorescence studies of Shope

papilloma virus in cottontail rabbit tissue cultures. *Proc. Soc. exp. Biol.* (New York) *128:* 1025

273 PANTELEAKIS, P. N., LARSON, V. M., GLENN, E. S., & HILLEMAN, M. R. (1968) Prevention of viral transplantable tumors in hamsters, employing killed and fragmented homologous tumor-cell vaccines. *Proc. Soc. exp. Biol.* (New York) *129:* 50

274 PAPADIMITRIOU, J. M. (1917) Ultrastructural features of chronic murine hepatitis after reovirus 3 infection. *Brit. J. exp. Path. 47:* 624

275 PARSONS, R. J., & KIDD, J. (1943) Oral papillomatosis of rabbits: a virus disease. *J. exp. Med. 77:* 233

276 PAYNE, L. N., & CHUBB, R. C. (1968) Studies on the nature and genetic control of an antigen in normal chick embryos which reacts in the COFAL test. *J. gen. Virol. 3:* 379

277 PERK, K., SHACHAT, D. A., & MOLONEY, J. B. (1968) Pathogenesis of a rhabdomyosarcoma in rats induced by a murine sarcoma virus. *Cancer. Res. 28:* 1197

278 PIKE, M. C., WILLIAMS, E. H., & WRIGHT, B. (1967) Burkitt's tumour in the West Nile district of Uganda, 1961–65. *Brit. Med. J. 2:* 395

279 PITELKA, D. R., BERN, H. A., NANDI, S., & DEOME, K. B. (1964) On the significance of virus particles in the mammary tissues of CH3f mice. *J. nat. Canc. Inst. 33:* 867

280 POPE, J. H. (1963) The isolation of a mouse leukaemia virus resembling Friend virus. *Austral. J. exp. Biol. med. Sci. 40:* 263 and *41:* 349

281 PORTER, G. H., DALTON, A. S., MOLONEY, J. B., & MITCHELL, E. Z. (1964) Association of electron-dense particles with human acute leukaemia. *J. nat. Canc. Inst. 33:* 547

282 POSTLETHWAITE, R. (1964) Antiviral activity in extracts from lesions of molluscum contagiosum. *Virology 22:* 508

283 POTTER, G. W., OXFORD, J. S., & HOSKINS, J. M. (1969) Immunological relationships of some oncogenic DNA-viruses. *Arch. ges Virusforsch. 27:* 87

284 PURDY, W. J. (1932) The propagation of the Rous sarcoma No. 1 in ducklings. *Brit. J. exp. Path. 13:* 473

285 RABIN, H. and SLADEN, W. J. L. (1969) Examination of various avian sera for neutralizing antibody and susceptibility to Rous virus. *Amer. J. Epidem. 89:* 325

286 RABOTTI, G. F., GROVE, A. S., SELLERS, R. L., & ANDERSON, W. R. (1966) Induction of multiple brain tumours in dogs by Rous sarcoma virus. *Prog. Med. Virol. 209:* 884. S. Kargen, Basel and New York

287 ——, SELLERS, R. L., & ANDERSON, W. R. (1966) Leptomeningeal sarcomata and gliomata induced in rabbits by Rous sarcoma virus. *Nature* (London) *209:* 524

288 RABSON, A. S., O'CONOR, G. T., BEREZESKY, I. K., & PAUL, F. J. (1964) Enhancement of adenovirus growth in African green monkey cell cultures by SV 40. *Proc. Soc. exp. Biol.* (New York) *116:* 187

289 RAFFERTY, K. A. (1964) Kidney tumors of the leopard frog: a review. *Cancer Res. 24:* 169

290 RAPP, F., KHERA, K. S., & MELNICK, J. L. (1964) Resistance of BHK21 hamster cells to SV 40 papovavirus. *Nature 201:* 1349

291 —— & MELNICK, J. L. (1966) Papovavirus SV 40, adenovirus and their hybrids: transformation, complementation and transcapsidation. *Progr. med. Virol. 8:* 349

292 ROGERS, S. (1952) Serial transplantation of rabbit papillomas caused by the Shope virus. *J. exp. Med. 95:* 543

293 —— & ROUS, P. (1951) Joint action of a chemical carcinogen and a neoplastic virus to induce cancer in rabbits. *Ibid. 93:* 459

294 ROSE, S. M., & ROSE, F. C. (1952) Tumor agent transformations in amphibia. *Cancer Res. 12:* 1

295 ROUS, P. (1911) A sarcoma of the fowl transmissible by an agent separable from the tumor cells. *J. exp. Med. 13:* 397

296 —— (1913) Resistance to a tumor-producing agent as distinct from resistance to the implanted tumor cells. *Ibid. 18:* 416

297 —— & BEARD, J. W. (1934) An induced mammalian growth with the characters of a tumor (the Shope rabbit papilloma). *Ibid. 60:* 701

298 —— & —— (1935) The progression to carcinoma of virus-induced papilloma (Shope). *Ibid. 62:* 523

299 ——, KIDD, J. G., & SMITH, W.C. (1938) The carcinogenic effect of a papilloma virus on the tarred skin of rabbits. *Ibid. 67:* 399 and 529

300 ——, ——, & —— (1952) Experiments on the cause of the rabbit carcinomas derived from virus-induced papillomas. 2. *Ibid. 96:* 159

301 —— & MURPHY, J. B. (1912) The histological signs of resistance to a transmissible sarcoma of the fowl. *Ibid. 15:* 270

302 —— & —— (1913) Variations in a chicken sarcoma caused by a filterable agent. *Ibid. 17:* 219

303 —— & —— (1914) On immunity to transplantable chicken tumors. *Ibid. 20:* 419

304 ——, ROBERTSON, O. H., & OLIVIA, J. (1919) Experiments on production of specific antisera for infections of unknown cause. 2. *Ibid. 29:* 305

305 —— & SMITH, W. C. (1945) The neoplastic potentialities of mouse embryo tissues. 1. *Ibid. 81:* 597

306 ROWE, W. P., & BAUM, S. G. (1964) Evidence for a possible genetic hybrid between adenovirus type 7 and SV 40. *Proc. nat. Acad. Sci.* (Washington) *52:* 1340

307 ——, HUEBNER, R. J., HARTLEY, J. W. (1961) Ecology of a mouse tumor virus. *Perspectives in virology 2:* 177. Burgess: Minneapolis

308 ROWSON, K. E. K., & MAHY, B. J. W. (1967) Human papova (wart) virus. *Bact. Rev. 31:* 110

309 ——, ROE, F. J. C., BALL, J. K., & SALAMAN, M. H. (1961) Induction of tumours by polyoma virus: enhancement by chemical agents. *Nature 191:* 893

310 RUBIN, H. (1956) An analysis of the apparent neutralization of Rous sarcoma virus with antisera to normal chick tissues. *Virology 2:* 545

311 ——, CORNELIUS, A., & FANSHIER, L. (1961) The pattern of congenital transmission of an avian leukosis virus. *Proc. nat. Acad. Sci.* (Washington) *47:* 1058

312 ——, FANSHIER, L., CORNELIUS, A., & HUGHES, W. F. (1962)

Tolerance and immunity in chickens after congenital and contact infection with an avian leukosis virus. *Virology 17:* 143

313 ——— & VOGT, P. K. (1962) An avian leukosis virus associated with stocks of Rous sarcoma virus. *Virology 17:* 184

314 RUSSELL, W. E., & KNIGHT, B. E. (1967) Evidence for a new antigen within the adenovirus capsid. *J. gen. Virol. 1:* 523

315 SABIN, A. B., & KOCH, M. A. (1963) Evidence of continuous transmission of SV 40 viral genome in most or all SV 40 hamster tumor cells. *Proc. nat. Acad. Sci.* (Washington) *49:* 304

316 ——— (1969) The search for a DNA-virus as an etiologic agent of human cancer. *Int. Virology 1:* 189

317 SARMA, P. S., TURNER, H. C., & HUEBNER, R. J. (1964) An avian leukosis group-specific complement-fixation reaction. *Virology 23:* 313

318 SCHÄFER, W., & ECKERT, E. A. (1968) Production of a potent complement-fixing murine leukemia virus antiserum from the rabbit. *Virology 35:* 323

319 SCHMIDT, N. J., KING, C. J., & LENNETTE, E. H. (1965) Haemagglutination and haemagglutinin-absorption with adenovirus type 12. *Proc. Soc. exp. Biol.* (New York) *118:* 208

320 SCHMIDT-RUPPIN, K. H. (1964) Hetero-transplantation of Rous sarcoma and Rous sarcoma virus to mammals. *Oncologia 17:* 247

321 SHEIN, H. M., ENDERS, J. F., PALMER, L., & GROGAN, E. (1964) Further studies on SV 40-induced transformation in human renal cell cultures. 1. *Proc. Soc. exp. Biol.* (New York) *115:* 618

322 SHIRATORI, O., OSATO, T., UTSUMI, R., & ITO, Y. (1968) Growth and other characteristics of a cell-line established from Shope virus-induced cutaneous papillomas in domestic rabbits. *Proc. Soc. exp. Biol.* (New York) *128:* 12

323 SHOPE, R. E. (1932) A filtrable virus causing a tumor-like condition in rabbits and its relationship to virus myxomatosis. *J. exp. Med. 56:* 803

324 ——— (1933) Infectious papillomatosis of rabbits. *Ibid. 58:* 607

325 ——— (1966) Evolutionary episodes in the concepts of viral oncogenesis. *Perspect. Biol. Med. 9:* 258

326 ———, MANGOLD, R., MACNAMARA, L. G., & DUMBELL, K. R. (1958) An infectious cutaneous fibroma of the Virginian white-tailed deer. *J. exp. Med. 108:* 797

327 SIMONS, P. J., DOURMASHKIN, R. R., TURANO, A., PHILLIPS, D. E. H., & CHESTERMAN, F. C. (1967) Morphological transformation of mouse embyro cells *in vitro* by murine sarcoma virus (Harvey). *Nature 214:* 897

328 ———, PEPPER, S. S., & BAKER, R. S. V. (1969) Different cell-culture characteristics of two strains of mouse sarcoma virus. *Proc. Soc. exp. Biol.* (New York) *131:* 454

329 SINKOVICS, J. G. (1962) Viral leukemia in mice. *Ann. Rev. Microbiol. 16:* 75

330 SJÖGREN, H. O., HELLSTROM, I., & KLEIN, G. (1961) Transplantation of polyoma-virus-induced tumors in mice. *Cancer Res. 21:* 329

331 SMITH, R. R., HUEBNER, R. J., ROWE, W. P., SCHATTEN, W. E., &

THOMAS, L. B. (1956) Studies on the use of viruses in the treatment of carcinoma of the cervix. *Cancer* (Philadelphia) *9:* 1211

332 SMITH, W. & MACKAY, J. M. K. (1969) Morphological observations on a virus associated with sheep pulmonary adenomatosis (jaagsiekte). *J. comp. Path. 79:* 421

333 SOUTHAM, C. M., & MOORE, A. E. (1962) Clinical studies of viruses as antineoplastic agents. *Cancer* (Philadelphia) *5:* 1025

334 STANLEY, N. F., & KEAST, D. (1967) A reovirus-specific antigen in murine lymphoma. *Aust. J. exp. Biol. med. Sci. 45:* 517

335 —— & —— (1967) Murine infection with reovirus 3 as a model for the virus induction of auto-immune disease and neoplasia. *Perspectives in Virology 5:* 281. Academic Press, New York and London

336 STEWART, S. E., & DURR, F. E. (1967) Brain lesions in experimental animals produced with an agent from Burkitt tumor cultures. *Perspectives in Virology 5:* 167. Academic Press, New York and London

337 ——, EDDY, B. E., & BORGESE, N. G. (1958) Neoplasms in mice inoculated with a tumor agent carried in tissue culture. *J. nat. Canc. Inst. 20:* 1223

338 STOKER, M. G. P. (1960) Studies on the oncogenic activity of the Toronto strain of polyoma virus. *Brit. J. Cancer 14:* 679

339 —— (1964) Regulation of growth and orientation in hamster cells transformed by polyoma virus. *Virology 24:* 165

340 (1966) General aspects of cell interaction with oncogenic viruses. In *Comparative leukemia research,* p. 1. Pergamon Press, Oxford

341 —— (1968) Abortive transformation by polyoma virus. *Nature* (London) *218:* 234

342 —— & RUBIN, H. Density-dependent inhibition of cell growth in culture. *Nature* (London) *215:* 171

343 —— & MACPHERSON, I. (1961) Studies on transformation of hamster cells by polyoma virus *in vitro. Virology 14:* 359

344 ——, O'NEILL, C., BERRYMAN S., & WAXMAN, V. (1968) Anchorage and growth regulation in normal and virus-transformed cells. *Int. J. Cancer 3:* 683

345 ——, SHEARER, M., & O'NEILL, C. (1966) Growth inhibition of polyoma-transformed cells by contact with static normal fibroblasts. *J. Cell Sci. 1:* 297

346 STRANDSTRÖM, H. V., AMBRUS, J. L., & OWENS, G. (1966) Propagation of Yaba virus in embryonated hen's eggs. *Virology 28:* 479

347 STÜCK, B. E., BOYSE, E. A., OLD, L. J., & CARSWELL, E. A. (1964) ML: a new antigen found in leukaemias and mammary tumors of the mouse. *Nature* (London) *203:* 1033

348 SVEC, F., ALTANER, C., & HLAVAY, E. (1966) Pathogenicity for rats of a strain of chicken sarcoma. *J. nat. Canc. Inst. 36:* 389

349 ——, HLAVAY, E., THURZO, V., & KOSSEY, P. (1957) Erythroleukämie des Ratte, hervorgerufen durch zellfrei Karzinom-Filtrate. *Acta haematol. 17:* 34

350 SVET-MOLDAVSKY, G. J., & SKORIKOVA, A. S. (1964) The pathogenicity of Rous sarcoma virus for mammals. *Acta virol.* (Prague) *4:* 47

351 ——, TRUBCHENINOVA, L., & RAVKINA, L. I. (1967) Pathogenicity

of the chicken sarcoma virus (Schmidt-Ruppin) for amphibians and reptiles. *Nature* (London) *214:* 300

352 SVOBODA, J. (1962) In *Mechanisms of immune tolerance,* p. 199. Academic Press, New York

353 —— & KLEMENT, V. (1963) Formation of delayed tumours in hamsters inoculated with Rous virus after birth. *Folia biol.* (Prague) *9:* 403

354 —— & SIMKOVIC, D. (1963) The relationships between virus and cell in rat sarcomas induced by Rous virus. *Acta un. int. Cancr. 19:* 302

355 SWEET, H., & HILLEMAN, M. R. (1960) The vacuolating agent SV 40. *Proc. Soc. exp. Biol.* (New York) *105:* 420

356 SYVERTON, J. T. (1952) The pathogenesis of the rabbit papilloma to carcinoma sequence. *Ann. N.Y. Acad. Sci. 54:* 1126

357 TEN SELDAM, R. E. J., COOKE, R. A., & ANDERSON, L. (1965) Childhood lymphomas in the territories of Papua and New Guinea. *Cancer* (Philadelphia) *19:* 437

358 THORBURN, M. T., GWYNN, A. V. R., RAGBEER, M. S., & LEE, B. I. (1968) Pathological and cytogenetic observations on the naturally occurring canine venereal tumour in Jamaica. *Brit. J. Cancer 22:* 720

359 TODARO, G. J., & BARON, S. (1965) The role of interferon in the inhibition of SV 40 transformation of mouse cell-line 3T3. *Proc. nat. Acad. Sci.* (Washington) *54:* 752

360 TRENTIN, J. J., YABE, Y., & TAYLOR, G. (1962) The quest for human cancer viruses . . . cancer induction in hamsters by human adenoviruses. *Science 137:* 825

361 TWEEDELL, K., & GRANOFF, A. (1968) Viruses and renal carcinomas of *Rana pipiens.* 5. *J. nat. Canc. Inst. 40:* 407

362 TYTLER, W. H. (1913) A transplantable new growth of the fowl producing cartilage and bone. *J. exp. Med. 17:* 466

363 VAAGE, J. (1968) Non-cross-reacting resistance to virus-induced mouse mammary tumours in virus-infected C3H mice. *Nature* (London) *218:* 101

364 —— (1969) Non-virus-associated antigens in virus-induced mouse mammary tumors. *Cancer Res. 28:* 2477

365 VIZOSO, A. D., HAY, R., & BATTERSBY, T. (1966) Isolation of unidentified agents capable of morphologically transforming hamster cells *in vitro. Nature* (London) *209:* 1263

366 VOGT, P. K. (1965) Avian tumor viruses. *Adv. Virus Res. 11:* 293

367 —— (1967) Non-producing state of Rous sarcoma cells. *J. Virol. 1:* 729

368 WEISS, D. W., BONHAG, R. S., & DEOME, K. B. (1961) Protective action of fractions of tubercle bacilli against isologous tumours in mice. *Nature 190:* 889

369 WOLFF, K. (1966) The fish viruses. *Adv. Virus Res. 12:* 35

370 YAMAMOUCHI, K., FUKUDA, A., KOBUNE, F., & UCHIDA, N. (1967) Oncogenicity of Schmidt-Ruppin strain of Rous sarcoma virus for cynomolgus monkeys. *Jap. J. med. Sci. Biol. 20:* 443

371 YOHN, D. S., HAMMON, W., McD., ATCHISON, R. W., & CASTO,

B. C. (1968) Oncogenic potentials of non-human viruses for human cancer. *J. nat. Canc. Inst. 41:* 523

372 ——, HAENDIGES, V. A., & GRACE, J. T. (1966) Yaba tumor pox virus synthesis *in vitro.* 1. *J. Bact. 91:* 1977

373 YOSHIDA, T. O., & ITO, Y. (1968) Immunofluorescent study on early virus–cell interaction in Shope papilloma *in vitro* system. *Proc. Soc. exp. Biol.* (New York) *128:* 587

374 YUILL, T. M., & HANSON, R. P. (1964) Infection of suckling cottontail rabbits with Shope's fibroma virus. *Proc. Soc. exp. Biol.* (New York) *117:* 376

375 ZILBER, L. A., & KRYUKOVA, I. N. (1957) Haemorrhagic diseases of rats caused by Rous sarcoma virus. *Probl. Virol.* (USSR) (Engl. transl.) *2:* 247

376 —— & SHELVLJAGHYN, V. (1964) Transformation of human embryonic cells by Rous sarcoma virus. *Nature* (London) *203:* 194

Glossary

Adenocarcinoma: a malignant tumour with gland-like structure.
Adenomatosis: presence of multiple tumours of gland-like structure.
Anaplasia (anaplastic): reversion to cells of more primitive nature.
Auto-immune disease: disease caused by formation of antibodies against constituents of an animal's own body.
Basophilia: having affinity for basic dyes.
Bursa of Fabricius: a collection of lymphoid tissue near the cloaca of fowls, having functions similar to that of the thymus in mammals.
Capsid: the rigid box enclosing the nucleoprotein of viruses with cubical symmetry.
Capsomeres: the protein subunits which together make up the capsid of a virus.
Carcinoma: a malignant tumour or cancer made of cells of epithelial origin; the word cancer is commonly used for any malignant tumour.
Carcinogenic (carcinogenesis): causing cancer.
Carrier-culture: see text p. 72.
Cellulitis: inflammation of connective tissue.
Cervix: neck, especially of uterus.
Cloning: separation of a line of genetically similar cells (or animals).
COFAL test: complement-fixation test for avian leukosis.
Collagen (collagenous): the main organic constituent of connective tissue.
Complement: a substance in serum recognized by its function in some immunological reactions such as lysis of red blood cells by antibody.
Complement fixation: a test for the presence of an antigen–antibody reaction by measuring the removal of complement from a system under study.
Complementation: the activity of a virus in restoring a defect which prevents another virus from multiplying.
Contact inhibition: see text p. 73.
Cytocidal: killing cells.
Cytopathic or **cytotoxic:** damaging cells.
Dalton: the unit of atomic weight.
Eosinophilic: having affinity for eosin or other acid dyes.
Epithelioid: resembling epithelium.
Epithelioma: a malignant tumour derived from epithelial cells, usually those of skin or mucous surfaces.
Erythroblastosis (erythrocytosis): excessive formation of red blood cells.
Erythroid: concerning the red blood cell system.
Erythropoietic: making red blood cells.

Feeder: see text p. 74.

Fibroma: an innocent tumour composed mainly of fibrous or developed connective tissue.

Fibrosarcoma: a malignant tumour derived from fibrous tissue.

Forsmann antigen: a protein present in organs of guinea pigs and other species: it can elicit antibodies which lyse sheep blood cells.

Genome: the genetic apparatus, comprising the whole complement of genes.

Granuloma: a tumour made up of granulation tissue.

Haemagglutinin: a substance which clumps red blood cells.

Haemopoietic: making blood cells.

HeLa and HEp: continuously propagated lines of cells derived from human carcinomata.

Helper: see text p. 27.

Hepatitis: inflammation of the liver.

Heterophile antibody test: one involving agglutination of sheep red cells.

Homograft: a graft of tissue from an animal of the same species.

Hyperplasia (hyperplastic): increase in number of tissue elements.

Icosahedron: a twenty-sided figure.

Immunological tolerance: failure of immunological response to an antigen; see text p. 22.

Inclusion body: a mass within cytoplasm or nucleus of a cell, often a response to a virus infection.

Interferon: a protein formed by cells, especially in response to a virus infection and having antiviral activity; see text p. 129.

Keratinized: rendered horny.

Kieselgühr: a diatomaceous earth.

Laparotomy: an operation involving opening the abdominal cavity.

Leukaemia: a malignant disease of blood-forming organs resulting in presence of large numbers of leukocytes or their precursors in the blood.

Leukosis: as for leukaemia but without there necessarily being excessive leukocytes in blood.

Lymphatic leukaemia: leukaemia involving the lymphocytic system.

Lymphoma (-atosis): a tumour made up of lymphoid tissue; if malignant it is a lymphosarcoma.

Lysogenic: a term applied to bacteria which may liberate a bacteriophage capable of lysing them or (more usually) other bacteria.

Macrophages: large phagocytic cells.

Metastases: secondary deposits of a malignant tumour.

Mutagen (mutagenic): able to cause mutations.

Mycoplasma: one of a family of small, often filterable, bacteria, formerly classed with the viruses.

Myeloblasts: primitive cells of the (myelocytic) series forming polymorphonuclear leukocytes.

Myeloid (myeloblastic) leukaemia: leukaemia involving cells of the myelocytic series.

Neoplasia: new growth or cancer; see text p. 5.

Neuraminidase: an enzyme which splits off sialic acid from a mucopolysaccharide.

Neuroblastoma: a tumour involving primitive nerve cells.

New growth: a tumour; see text p. 5.

nm.: one thousandth of a micron or 1 metre $\times 10^{-9}$ (same as 1 mμ).

Nucleocapsid: the nucleic acid of a virus together with the protein sub-units associated with it.

Nucleoid: a dense nucleus-like body in the centre of a virion.

Oncogenic: able to cause tumours.

Oncology (oncologist): study (student) of tumours.

Osteochondrosarcoma: a malignant tumour containing elements of bone and cartilage.

Osteosarcoma: a malignant tumour containing elements of bone.

Papilloma: a benign tumour or wart.

Papovavirus: see text p. 64.

Passenger: a virus present in or carried along in transplanted tumours or other tissues but having no causative role.

Phenotypical: not genetically determined nor heritable.

Pleomorphic: having various forms.

Pseudotype: virus having characters determined by the presence of an outer coat which may be changed for one of different origin.

Pyknotic: condensed.

Reversion (revertant): a term used of transformed cells which revert to normal.

Rhabdomyosarcoma: a malignant growth containing elements derived from striped muscles.

Sarcoma: a malignant growth of connective tissue origin.

Serotype: a strain of an organism distinguished from others by specific serological characters.

Superinfection: a second infection imposed on one already present.

Thymectomy: excision of the thymus gland.

Transformation: a change occurring in tissue culture, so that it has some of the characters of malignancy; see text p. 72.

Transplantation antigen: one concerned in the rejection of grafts of tumours or other tissues; see text p. 82.

Vacuolation: formation of vesicles or cavities.

Vertical transmission: transmission of an agent from members of one generation to its descendants.

Viraemia: presence of virus in the blood.

Virion: the mature form of a virus in which it is normally transmitted from one host to another.

Index

A particles, 43
Abortive transformation, 78, 84
Accelerating factors, 2, 52, 99
Adenocarcinoma, 17, 44, 64, 99
Adenomatosis, pulmonary, 93, 95, plate 20
Adenosine triphosphatase, 20, 21, 49
Adenoviruses, 9, 10, 11, 68–71, 80, 82, 84, 125, 137, plates 15, 16
Africa, 93, 104–7
Age and cancer, 67, 104, 126, 127
AKR mice, 46, 51, 52, 99
Antibody, see Neutralization, Gel-diffusion, Complement-fixation
Anti-lymphocytic serum, 129
Antigenic differences, 13, 28, 45
Arboviruses, 11, 106, 111, 122, 124
Autonomy, 51

B particles, 41, 43, 44
Base-ratios, 11, 69
BCG, 138
BHK 21 cells, 73
Bryan strain of Rous virus, 29
Bunyamwera virus, 124
Bursa of Fabricius, 23
Burkitt tumour, 25, 104–11, 136, plates 23, 24

C particles, 48, 59–62, 136, plate 11
Cancer houses, 138
Canine tumour, 133–4
Capsid (and capsomeres), 10, 11, 64, 68, 86, 136, plate 1
Carcinogenic compounds, 5, 12–16, 130

Carcinoma in situ, 138
Carr-Zilber virus, 34, 36
Carrier culture, 72, 73, 77
Cattle, 60–2, 89
Cebus monkey, 90, 97
Cell-mediated immunity, 83, 96
Cercopithecus monkey, 67, 70, 97, 108, 109
Cervical cancer, 125, 134, 135
Chemotherapy, 104
Chicken, see Fowl
Chimpanzee, 108, 109
Chorio-allantoic membrane, 16, 98
Chromosomes, 25, 30, 76, 78, 107, 128, 134
Clusters, 60, 61, 138
COFAL test, 29, 37, 38
Complement, 16
Complementation, 70
Complement-fixation, 37, 108, 136
Conditional infections, 1, 2
Contact-inhibition, 28, 73, 82
Cortisone (and related substances), 116, 119, 120
Cotton-rat, 36
Cotton-tail, 4, 85–7, 96, 115
Crisis, 79
Cross-reactions, 15, 29, 45, 49, 82, 129
Cynomolgus monkey, 37, 108
Cytomegalovirus, 129
Cytotoxic (tests, etc.), 49, 54, 80, 82, 127

Deer, 58, 89
Defective viruses, 27, 28, 29, 56, 135

Density-dependent inhibition, 74
Deoxyuridines, 20
'Disappearance' of virus, 76, 90, 93
DNA, 8, 10, 11, 49, 64, 67, 76, 77, 86, 88, 102
DNA-viruses, 8, 10, 25, 63, 72, 76, 86, 101
Dogs, 36, 68, 89, 133–4
Ducks, 32–4

Early proteins, 81, 137
EB virus, 61, 106–10, 136
Encephalitis, 125
Erythroblastosis, 21, 53–4

Feeder, 74, 110
Fibre, 68, 69, 77
Fibrosarcoma, 64, 66, 67, 116
Filament, 64, 86
Fibroma of rabbits, 2, 4, 94–7, 114–16
Filtration, 12, 14, 27, 37, 60
Fish, 102–3
Fluorescent, see Immunofluorescence
Forssman antigen, 20
Foster-nursing, 39
Fowl paralysis, 19
Fowl pox, 2, 94, 118
Fowl tumour, 3, 4, 6, 9, 12–38, 113, plates 3, 4, 5, 6
Friend virus, 48, 52–4, 56, 130
Frog, 25, 99–101
Fujinami virus, 16, 32
Fusion of cells, 35, 77, 128

Gel-diffusion, 107
Genetic differences, 25, 26, 30, 40
Germ-free animals, 48
Goose, 15
Graffi virus, 48, 54
Graft, see Host reaction
Gross, virus, 46–9, 51–2, 54, 131
Guinea fowl, 32, 33
Guinea pig, 34, 58–9

Haemagglutinin, 10, 64, 69
Haemorrhagic disease, etc., 16, 34, 36
Hamster, chinese, 34, 36
Hamster, golden or Syrian, 34, 35, 51, 56, 66, 67, 73, 80, 89, 135
Hamster, spontaneous tumours, 62, 134
Hare, 95, 97
HeLa (and HEp) cells, 68
Helper, 6, 27, 33, 38, 56
Herpesviruses, 9, 10, 25, 61, 100, 106, 107, 112, 129, 134, 135, 137, plates 1, 12
Hexon, 68
Hormones, 1, 40, 41
Host reaction, 110
Horses, 89
Human cells, 78–9, 123
Hybridization, 70–1

Immunization, 44, 82, 84
Immunofluorescence, 80, 81, 86, 87, 107
Immunological tolerance, 22, 34, 44, 50, 83
Immunological surveillance, 126–7
Inclusion bodies, 10, 25, 88, 98, 99, plate 2
Infectious mononucleosis, 108, 110
Inhibitors, 41
Initiation, 3, 129, 130
Integration, 63, 78
Interferon, 61, 120

Jaagsiekte, 93, plate 20

Kidney grafts, 129
Kidney tumours, 17, 44, 65, 96, 99–101

Lepus, 90, 95
Leukaemia (leukosis) in cattle, 60–1; in cats, 59–60; in dogs, 60; in fowls, 5, 12, 18–23; in guinea